Ethics
The Heart of Health Care

Third Edition

David Seedhouse

Auckland University of Technology, New Zealand
Staffordshire University, UK
South Staffordshire and Shropshire Healthcare NHS Foundation Trust
Values Exchange: www.values-exchange.com

WILEY-BLACKWELL

A John Wiley & Sons, Ltd., Publication

Values
EXCHANGE
A VOICE FOR EVERYONE

This edition first published 2009
© 1988, 1998, 2009 John Wiley & Sons

Wiley-Blackwell is an imprint of John Wiley & Sons, formed by the merger of Wiley's global Scientific, Technical and Medical business with Blackwell Publishing.

Registered office
John Wiley & Sons Ltd, The Atrium, Southern Gate, Chichester, West Sussex, PO19 8SQ, United Kingdom

Editorial office
John Wiley & Sons Ltd, The Atrium, Southern Gate, Chichester, West Sussex, PO19 8SQ, United Kingdom

For details of our global editorial offices, for customer services and for information about how to apply for permission to reuse the copyright material in this book please see our website at www.wiley.com/wiley-blackwell.

Library of Congress Cataloging-in-Publication Data

Seedhouse, David, 1956–
   Ethics : the heart of health care / David Seedhouse. – 3rd ed.
      p. ; cm.
   Includes bibliographical references and index.
   ISBN 978-0-470-01813-2 (pbk.)
  1. Medical ethics. I. Title.
   [DNLM: 1. Ethics, Clinical. 2. Ethics, Medical. WB 60 S451e 2008]
   R724.S4325 2008
   174'.2–dc22
                                 2008032239

A catalogue record for this book is available from the British Library.

Set in 10 on 12 pt Sabon by SNP Best-set Typesetter Ltd., Hong Kong
Printed in Singapore by Markono Print Media Pte Ltd

1 2009

Contents

The colour plate section can be found between pages 164 and 165.

ABOUT THE AUTHOR

David Seedhouse was born in Nottingham, England. He was educated (a little) at Carre's Grammar School, Sleaford (1967–74), then a little more at Manchester University (1977–84), though mostly he taught himself.

David has written or edited 14 books (including second and third editions) and was founding editor of the journal *Health Care Analysis*. Despite this scholarly success, David turned his back on an academic career, choosing instead to create and market web-based decision-support tools based on his philosophical ideas.

David's main business products are the Values Exchange: www.values-exchange.com – and the Health Exchange: http://hx.values-exchange.co.uk/about/abouthx.aspx. Currently there are 22 Values Exchanges and two Health Exchanges – owned by NHS Trusts, universities and schools. David predicts a rapid expansion in the take-up of these products.

David moved to Auckland in 1992 and is a citizen of both Britain and New Zealand. Today he spends an increasing amount of time in the UK, developing and promoting his unique business. David is married to Hilary, with whom he is raising two daughters, Charlotte – a talented writer – and Penelope – a comic genius.

David can be contacted at david@values-exchange.com.

Preface to the Third Edition

The conceptually inadequate culture of conventional health care has hardly changed at all since I wrote the first edition of this book. The medical system continues to confuse clinical technique with health work; 'ethicists' tell clinical students they must obey moral rules and principles if they want to be ethical; and countless opportunities to improve health go begging every day because most health professionals don't reflect deeply enough on the purpose of their work.

Health and medical ethics texts – this one included – will never change this situation.

But this is no reason to despair – change takes time and time brings fresh opportunity. Today the ideas contained in the first two editions have been turned into software which is increasingly being used in health care training and practice.

Most people who use the Values Exchange (www.values-exchange.com) will never read *Ethics: The Heart of Health Care* nor realise they are thinking philosophically as they respond to its cases – but that is the way of the world. When we fly few of us think about research on jet propulsion, but we benefit from it having been done.

When I wrote the Preface to the first edition I sincerely believed that if enough people read my book, the world would change. When I wrote the Preface to the second edition I had found out that reading books is never enough to change the world – I even went so far as to urge health workers to put their ethics books away. I encouraged them to think deeply for themselves instead, and I hoped they would commit personally to a compassionate philosophy of health.

Now I have learnt that this is asking too much too. People have lives full to overflowing, most do not find philosophical thinking easy, and many prefer to read advice from 'ethics experts' because they don't have the time or experience to think the complexities through independently.

Now I know what doesn't work. But I also know we all have philosophy and passion in us. With just a bit of support and encouragement we can be amazingly deep and thoughtful. So, this time round I am asking us to recognise the brilliance of the rational fields we create whenever we decide to do or change anything – this time I urge you to read this book; then quickly put it down, then think, then act to make the world better if you possibly can. Do so on your own terms, do so on the terms of those you are trying to help, do so on my terms, do so on the Values Exchange www.values-exchange.com – it doesn't matter so long as you feel and think and recognise inside the need to commit to an ethical way of being.

Preface to the Second Edition

If you are a health worker and you want to understand ethics you have two choices. You can study texts which take ethical principles for granted, or you can read books inspired by a theory of health. Both types discuss practical cases, but with a profound difference.

If you plump for 'principles first' books you step into quicksand. Different texts espouse conflicting axioms. Read enough and you'll find ethical principles behind every practice. Pro- and anti-abortion lobbies both have ethics on their side. There's a school of thought that considers health care rationing morally abhorrent, and another that thinks efficient resource allocation is what ethics is all about. Some societies claim that health services are morally special, others believe they sell commodities like any other business.

How do you choose between contrasting moral allegiances? And how do you respond to colleagues who do not hold your ethical beliefs? If they are utilitarian while you feel duty-bound to offer everyone equal care, how do you argue with them? If they insist they are right you'll never change their minds by just telling them they aren't.

You can escape the stalemate if you have a theory of health. If you do, your reasoning need not start with blind moral faith but with careful deliberation about the *point* of working for health in practical situations.

If you share the philosophy of health that informs *Ethics: The Heart of Health Care* then your moral outlook is not a purely intellectual matter either. If you choose to uphold this philosophy you make a commitment born of centuries of compassionate practice. And once you've made it you no longer have to barter principles. It is pointless to protest – 'this practice is unethical'. However, a practically relevant justification is essential:

> Excuse me doctor/nurse/manager/policy-maker, but what are you trying to achieve here? What is the purpose of your intervention? What inspires your behaviour?

If you get an answer you can debate fundamentals – not ethical whims. What notion of health does the response suggest? What would happen if the idea were applied consistently to all health work? Where does this understanding of health goals differ from your own? *Is* yours better? Why?

Because work for health is a moral endeavour it must be thoughtful. And because careful thinking matters so much it is not acceptable that health care decision-makers hide behind status, codes of practice, ethical biases dressed up as truths, or even the law. Whenever you ask – *how does what you are doing create better health?* – nothing less than honest, reasoned answers will do. This book will help you get them.

Preface to the First Edition

This book extends a theory about the nature of health into the heart of practice. It is genuinely philosophy applied. And it is long overdue.

In the majority of areas of human activity there exist theories, sometimes a range of competing theories, about the meaning of a particular activity, about its limits, about the sorts of methods and techniques that are most suited to it, about its implications for other areas of activity, and about the moral issues that are raised by it. Such theories are usually known as philosophies. So not only are there specific human activities known as medicine and social science, for instance, but there are also branches of inquiry which try to analyse and understand the rationale of the practices.

Thus there is a philosophy of medicine and a philosophy of social science which aim at uncovering the raison d'etre of each discipline. Since the philosophies are concerned with the underlying reasons for the practical activities so they inevitably have an influence on the future development of them.

Work within the philosophy of medicine may ask, for instance, whether treatments in medicine should be given at any cost, or whether there are occasions on which it is better not to treat patients. The philosophy of social science asks questions about what forms of inquiry are truly to count as social science, and about how much faith can be placed in the reliability of any results generated from inquiry in social science. The answers offered in response to such theoretical questions can have immense practical impact on the parent activities.

It is, at first sight, puzzling that there is no discipline concerned with the philosophy of health. Given that health work periodically affects every member of society (at least in the Western world) from a time before birth until death it is surprising that so little attention has been given to its philosophy. A partial explanation for this phenomenon is that 'health work' is a term with such a wide variety of meanings and applications – from open-heart surgery to political action over environmental hazards – that it is extremely difficult to identify it as a single coherent body of activity. Also, many of the constituent parts of health work – such as medicine and social science – already have their own philosophies.

However, it has been shown (Seedhouse 1986) that health work can be delineated – albeit within a broad boundary – and that this process of delineation and clarification can have implications for practice. For instance, some forms of practice – say, drug trials carried out on patients without their knowledge – can be seen to be work for health in only a very limited sense, if at all. And other practices not normally considered to be work for health – say, talking to a person to help him picture his social circumstances in a more realistic way – can now be seen to be work for health in a very strong sense. Clarification can change the priorities of practice.

Ethics: The Heart of Health Care further pioneers the exploration of the philosophy of health. By charting the extent to which moral issues permeate work for health, by demonstrating tangibly and graphically that work for health is truly a moral endeavour, a solid and useful theoretical basis for health workers of all kinds is created. From this platform health workers can grasp more firmly the theoretical significance of their everyday activities. Having gained a stronger grasp on theory health workers are placed in a far better position to appreciate the extent to which they have a huge personal responsibility for the health care they give. Such responsibility is frequently demanding and trying, but if it is handled with confidence it can also be exciting and fulfilling.

The argument of the book – philosophy applied

It is time that philosophy is again recognised for what it is. Philosophy is an essential part of the way in which we understand our world. It is a process of inquiry that can have real practical effect. The best philosophers are not happy merely to 'watch the wheels turn'. They know that what they do can help produce better wheels, or even rearrange those wheels so that a different machine is created. Philosophy can rejuvenate practice.

This book makes the following points and connections. It forms a powerful guide for those in health care who wish to work with a high degree of morality, and who would also like to improve the structure and organisation of health care. The world of health care is undergoing a period of intellectual crisis, quite separate from the current political and economic debates on the funding and cost-effectiveness of the NHS. There are a number of forces that are challenging existing assumptions and patterns of practice. These forces include rising interest in holistic medicine; increasing pressure by lay people to have access to medical secrets, including their own medical records; pressure to include the study of medical ethics in undergraduate curricula; and the arguments of some social scientists and health promoters that work for health must begin in society rather than focus on individuals. The tension between old and new ideas can be illustrated by an idea borrowed from the philosophy of science – the notion of 'paradigm shift'. It is best to think of this notion only as an analogy rather than a reality. The old paradigm – the old set of cherished beliefs and principles – is being called into question by the new forces. Hence a period of crisis exists in which conflicting ideas and principles do metaphorical battle.

The process of change from one paradigm to another is not definite and predictable. The future must, to an extent, be shaped actively by people. The question is: How is it possible to ensure that the new era of health care that emerges from the period of crisis has the best possible form and content? The route to an answer is opened up by offering health workers a more comprehensive understanding of the nature of ethics. Ethics is the key to the new era of health care. Health workers must know that work for health is a moral endeavour. But work for health is not a moral endeavour in the sense of a crusade. It is not a moral endeavour in an evangelical sense. The task is not to identify what is good and bad, right and wrong, as a dogmatist might. Ethics is not a discipline in which pure blacks and whites can be uncovered and then applied for ever without further question. Ethics is always a question of degree, a question of deliberating about which interventions in other people's lives will produce the highest possible degree of morality. But how can the degree of morality of an intervention be assessed in any objective sense? Both ethics and health work are beset by the problem that people in complex societies have different values and beliefs.

What one person believes to be a good intervention in the life of another, an intervention exhibiting a high degree of morality, another person might regard as a poor intervention. Even advice about diet and exercise is never based wholly on fact. At some stage a value judgement of some kind will be made.

The extent of the influence of value judgement can be seen from the case studies presented in Chapter Three (third edition). There are no clear-cut solutions to any of the situations presented, and whatever solution is proposed must involve some reference to values. Since people's values frequently conflict, how, if at all, can a firm theoretical basis for consistent moral intervention be given to which all health workers can assent?

There is a range of answers which fail.

1 One might search for the 'objectively good'. In other words one might pursue some ultimate value or ordering of values which is truly moral. But there can be no means of uncovering the 'truly moral' since in ethics much depends upon personal opinion and subjective judgement. It is not possible to discover the 'objectively good' as one might discover Mount Everest, or a solution to a problem in applied mathematics.
2 Alternatively, one might search for a set of rules, or a code of practice, to provide a firm uncontroversial basis. However, experience shows that whatever rule, or set of rules, is selected there are always exceptions. There will always be courses of action which offend the rules but lead to the creation of a higher degree of morality than if the rules had been obeyed.
3 One might appeal to law, but a similar problem to that of the appeal to rules arises.
4 Or one might instead settle for a relativist position, where it is accepted that there is no objective standard of morality, where what is to be done depends upon judgements made at the time under the existing circumstances. The trouble with this option is that morality can become a meaningless term. Given sufficient advocacy any form of intervention might become permissible for a time. Current law might prohibit some actions, but the higher court of appeal – the court of morality – will be left powerless.

Where is the foundation for consistent moral intervention to be found? An appeal has to be made to the facts about human nature and potential. Although it is very hard to determine what a truly good human potential or action is, it is less difficult to establish which actions are truly bad. It can be shown that certain ways of limiting human beings – ways of dwarfing people mentally, physically, and spiritually – are plainly immoral.

Consequently, moves to prevent dwarfing, examples of attempts to liberate the enhancing potentials that people possess, form a basis for the most moral health work.

How can this assertion be given support? Attention has to be paid to the definition of 'personhood'. What is a person, and what forms of human potential, out of all the possibilities, are the most important and significant? The view is advanced that the mental life of a person, which forms an essential part of the definition of 'personhood', is at least as important a target for health work as a person's physical life. It is important that health workers are in a position to apply the results of this analysis. So, with relevant and accessible examples, traditional theories of moral philosophy are explained. Too often in the past these theories have been left to languish in a scholarly vacuum. However, even with this theoretical background and firm base, there remains much uncertainty and room for conflicts of values within the ethics of health. But this is simply the nature of ethics. The right course of action cannot be prescribed as if it were a pill for a specific ill. There will always be legitimate alternative courses of action that might be chosen. Because of this constant need for deliberation and balancing of principles, a tool – the Ethical Grid – is offered to health workers both as an illustration of the nature of moral reasoning and as an aid to choosing actions to produce the highest degree of morality. Through the use of this tool health workers have the means to justify their choices, to explain how these choices might be shown to be the most strongly opposed to dwarfing.

The Ethical Grid is not a calculating machine. It is merely a euphemism for 'ethical reflection'. It can produce different solutions to the same situation dependent upon who is using it (that is to say, dependent upon who is deliberating). But it does enable health workers to be clear about what is immoral by indicating the range of interventions which lie beyond the limits of the grid. And by giving a clear core rationale the grid allows health workers a basis on which to decide for themselves between alternative possible interventions. Finally, recalling the ideas of crisis, paradigm change, and ethics as a key, some implications for the future of health care are considered. Principles such as 'respect for autonomy' and 'respect people as equals' have become likely new priorities for health work. If these principles, and others contained within the core of the grid, are accepted by those with the power to alter the shape of health care, then it will take on a different form. One possible new structure amongst many alternatives is sketched out to show how philosophical investigation – the process of clarification coupled with proposals generated out of logical analysis – can carry true practical weight.

Here, at last, are the beginnings of a philosophy of health.

Green Park
London, UK
September 1987

Acknowledgements

Time passes. Everything changes and everything stays the same.

I have had to squeeze this book into a busy software and business development schedule, and occasionally I thought I'd never get it done. The fact that I have – and whatever good and bad ideas it contains – are pretty much entirely my responsibility.

But I would like to thank Hilary for her support and resolve, Charlotte and Penny (and Jessica Tansey, their best friend) for being so alive, my development team for being brilliant and taking endless burdens from me, and Wiley for being patient and understanding of my changed circumstances.

Dates not yet mentioned: 25 October 1999, 12 November 2002 and 30 November 2006.

Dedication

For Simon and Mary Elstow

Introduction to the Third Edition

What this Third Edition is About

My first book, *Health: The Foundations for Achievement*, explained that health is a far richer concept than most people think (Figure 1).

My second book – the First Edition of *Ethics: The Heart of Health Care* – built on this holistic idea.

1 It introduced an Ethical Grid designed to help health workers think deeply and systematically about their daily practice
2 It argued that 'working for health' and 'creating morality' are necessarily related
3 It claimed that 'working for health' is as close to being objectively moral as it is possible to be.

Though the Ethical Grid has been used successfully by a generation of health educators, its philosophical development in the earlier editions was inadequate. Consequently, I no longer advocate points 2 and 3 in this Third Edition. Point 2 is too vague and 3 is completely wrong – there is no such thing as objective morality, so it is impossible to get close to it.

False assumptions

As in previous editions, the book begins by setting out four widely held but false assumptions. These are:

1 Health is the opposite of disease.
2 Health work is done solely to prevent, cure or alleviate the symptoms of disease.
3 Health work and medical care are identical activities.
4 Health work is what medically trained people do – no more and no less.

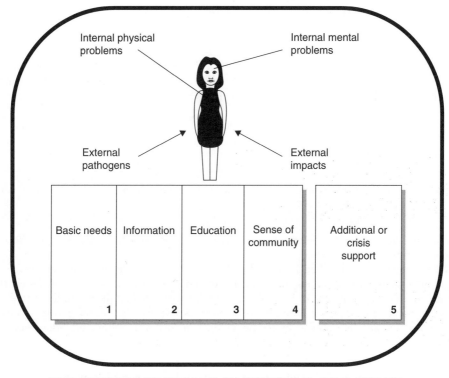

THE STATE OF HEALTH OF AN INDIVIDUAL OR A GROUP

Figure 1 All factors – including the social environment – must be included when assessing the health of the figure on the platform

These assumptions are incorrect because:

• Health can be defined in several ways other than 'the opposite of disease'.
• Therefore, medical care and health work are not necessarily the same.

Fortunately not all health workers are deceived:

1 Many health workers practice according to richer-than-clinical concepts of health.
2 As this trend grows – which one day it will – we will see a shift from a health care paradigm (**X**) dominated by technical priorities, to a health care paradigm (**Y**) where practical ethical reflection is as much a part of health care as clinical skill.

This book continues to hold that:

3 Genuine health interventions must always be attempts to liberate desirable human potential.
4 The richest health work aims to liberate the broadest range of human potentials, rather than focusing exclusively on disease and illness.
5 Attempting to liberate desirable human potential is the essence of morality.
6 Therefore, if morality means anything, genuine health work is quintessentially moral work.

However, *Ethics: The Heart of Health Care* (2008) recognises that things are quite a bit more complicated than they seemed in previous editions, and certainly move complex than I believed while writing the Preface to the First Edition.

The truth is not so simple

In 1988 and 1998 (to a lesser extent) I was captivated by what I felt to be a simple truth:

Just as (liberating desirable potential) is the true nature of work for health so it is also the true nature of moral endeavour . . .
    What is the point of mending a broken leg? What is the point of helping a person overcome emotional trauma through counselling? What is the point of trying to cure cancer? Surely the point is to enable each person to achieve more of whatever potential she has to live a fulfilled life. The point of eliminating obstacles to potential is not just that we judge the obstacles undesirable *per se*, the point is to get rid of them in order to release the good they are blocking.[1]

Health work removes obstacles to potential. The best health work removes the broadest range of obstacles – and so liberates the broadest range of potentials. The more desirable potential released, the more morality there is. It is a compelling idea.
    What's more, I thought I could actually demonstrate this relationship, using specific health examples, in a way with which no-one could possible disagree:

The first situation

A young man has been playing soccer and, during a hopelessly optimistic attempt at an overhead kick, has landed awkwardly and broken his left wrist. He does not know he has a broken bone but is in great pain and so visits the casualty department. On reporting to reception he is told in an unfriendly way to sit and wait his turn. He asks how long he will have to wait, but the receptionist tells him she has no idea. He then eats a packetful of boiled sweets. Three-quarters of an hour later he is approached by a nurse who conducts him to a small windowless room in which the doctor is sitting. The doctor does not look directly at the young man but focuses on the wrist, which he examines. He mumbles a few questions and then sends the patient to X-ray. The young man asks whether the bone is broken, and whether he need be in such pain. The doctor just shrugs, and tells him not to be a baby.

Even though he has now had a local anaesthetic, still the pain persists, and by now the young man is becoming anguished and fearful. He tells the doctor he is still in as much pain as ever, but the doctor does not believe him and, ignoring his protests, begins to set the wrist. This causes the patient excruciating agony. He screams involuntarily and is held down by three nurses until the doctor has done his work. After further pain and screams the doctor is satisfied. Without a word to the young man – of either explanation or apology – he leaves and a plaster cast is placed on the wrist by a surly technician. An appointment is made for the young man to return in 2 days' time, to check that the broken bone is still in the right place. He is advised to take paracetamol for the pain and to rest. Nothing else.

An alternative

The same young man has been playing football and has broken his left wrist. He visits the casualty department. On reporting to reception he is treated with kindness and sympathy. The receptionist, noting that the young man appears to be suffering a degree of shock, asks him how he is feeling and would he like to call anyone, and then invites him to sit and wait for the nurse, who will attend him as soon as she has seen patients who arrived before him – this will probably be in half an hour or so. The receptionist asks the young man whether he has eaten or drunk for the last 12 hours (it is now around mid-afternoon) and he replies that his last meal was supper yesterday. The receptionist explains that in this case it is best that he not eat anything now since it might just be that he will need a general anaesthetic, but that there is nothing at all to be alarmed about . . .

. . . the doctor organises the administration of a general anaesthetic. The bone is set.

When the young man regains consciousness a nurse sits with him until he feels well enough for his friend to drive him home. She explains about the visits he will have to make to the hospital in the future, about how quickly the pain will subside and about how soon he could expect to play football again.

What do these two situations indicate?

These situations go some way toward establishing the claim that work for health is a moral endeavour. They show that even in apparently routine health interventions, the manner in which a person is treated (and health produced) is inevitably bound up with the degree of morality created. Quite different physical, emotional and intellectual consequences might have been experienced by the young man, dependent upon how the health workers chose to act.

The key question for health workers is 'How can I intervene to the highest moral degree?' This question unites work for health with morality. It should be the permanent starting point for all health work.[2]

I still think, 'How can I intervene to the highest moral degree?' should be the first and last question every health worker asks, but, as I realised in the earlier editions:

Unfortunately, though this key question can be inspiring, it is so general that it is uninformative. For some people 'being ethical' means always conforming to a particular view about what is right and wrong. But when two people hold conflicting opinions about right and wrong in particular circumstances (as often happens) then their choices will conflict. Different people can have divergent ideas about how to intervene to the highest moral degree.

Considering that all involved are supposed to be working for health, such conflict is remarkably common in medicine . . . morality seems relative and contestable . . . competing views irreconcilable, and the idea of intervening morally open to almost any interpretation.

But this is not necessarily so. . . . Consider again the two situations above. In both cases effort aimed at creating health in the young man produced some degree of morality. The way to work out which behaviours generated the highest degree of morality is to note the extent to which the various aspects of the young man, thought of as a person rather than merely as a human body with a broken wrist, were repaired, enhanced, or developed.

Even in the down-to-earth setting of a casualty department there were opportunities to carry out very different sorts of intervention. In both situations the wrist was set. But in the first it was fixed with great and unnecessary pain, and the young man suffered uncertainty and anxiety: partly as a result of the receptionist's failure to inform him not to eat the boiled sweets, partly because he was not listened to by other staff, and because nothing of significance was explained to him. In the second situation attention was paid to his physical comfort, and time spent to enable him to understand his temporarily disabled circumstances and the future development of his wrist. He was also helped to feel emotionally calm and generally safe.

It is surely not unreasonable to conclude provisionally . . . that the interventions which took place in the second situation were of a higher moral standard than those which took place in the first.[3]

I firmly believed that anyone would judge the second situation to be more moral than the first, even though I knew simultaneously that the: 'key question ("How can I intervene to the highest moral degree?") . . . is so general that it is uninformative'.[3]

The Third Edition continues to take the view that health work and morality are related, but it is less philosophically naive. Obviously, not everyone will share my moral preferences, even if they share a commitment to the foundations theory of health. Even people with very similar general outlooks can and do justify contrasting choices about social situations – as the notorious 'Ashley Therapy' case illustrates.

The 'Ashley Therapy'

Ashley was born in 1997. Her cognitive function is equivalent to an infant's; she will never talk or walk, and is wholly dependent on her parents.

In 2004, after scrutiny by an Ethics Committee of around 40 members, Ashley's parents gained approval for the surgical removal of her uterus and breast buds. In addition, her doctors were permitted to administer high doses of oestrogen to retard her growth and sexual development, in order to enable her parents to continue to care for her indefinitely.[4]

Ashley stopped growing aged 9. Her 'treatment' is now complete, which means she will remain 4 feet 6 inches tall all her life.

The 'Ashley Therapy' has polarised commentators. In my opinion, short of gratuitous torture, her 'treatment' was just about as immoral as it gets – I believe she was deliberately and unnecessarily 'dwarfed' (see p. 270). I do not think her 'treatment' was health work because it restricted some of her central human potentials.

But other observers, just as passionate as I, disagree. For example, Dr Diekema, the spokesperson for the 40-strong ethics committee, gave the following answers when interviewed by CNN (http://edition.cnn.com/2007/HEALTH/01/11/ashley.ethicist/index. html), posted 11 January 2007:

Diekema: There were two main aspects to the parents' requests. We looked at whether we should permit growth attenuation to occur and whether we should permit a hysterectomy. The first issue was, do these things have the potential to improve this little girl's quality of life? Will they make her life better? And the second issue was, what's the potential for harm here and is it significant [enough] that even with the prospect of some benefit we shouldn't allow it to move forward? It was the consensus of the committee this did in fact actually have potential to improve her life significantly and there was very little actual harm.

CNN: As a doctor and an ethicist, what was most troubling to the ethics panel?

Diekema: The ethics committee struggled with trying to understand what potential troubles might come to a little girl from this sort of thing. Would someone in Ashley's position, for example, ever really care if they were 12 inches shorter? The conclusion was in Ashley's circumstances, where she would never walk or talk, that height had very little value. We needed to look at the different meaning these sorts of things might have to a little girl who is as profoundly disabled as Ashley was.

CNN: You pledge to do no harm, but this was the first case of its kind. How do you proceed knowing it was without precedent?

Diekema: One of the difficult things about being a physician is sometimes you don't know for sure. We strive to do no harm, but that has to be balanced against what good you might do for a patient. Ashley had a surgical procedure and that involves some pain and risk, but it was our assessment after very careful consideration that the potential benefits would ultimately outweigh the risks.

CNN: What are the benefits for Ashley?

Diekema: When you look at the growth attenuation, the primary benefits are by being a smaller girl, it will be easier for people to lift her, and will allow her to receive a more personal level of care from her parents for a longer period of time. They really want to be able to pick up their daughter and give her a hug and put her in a chair. ... As far as removing her uterus with a hysterectomy, there are many profoundly disabled children who are traumatized by menstruation. They don't understand why there is blood coming from that part of their body, and it's impossible to make them understand. Unlike a normal 11- or 12-year-old, you can't explain to them this is a normal part of your development. The family wanted to spare Ashley that drama. Ashley's a little girl who already had experienced being terrified of blood.

CNN: Ashley goes to school. She has peers. Is it at all concerning to you that here's a little girl who will never grow?

Diekema: It would be more concerning to me if she were a little girl who was running around on the playground. I think ultimately being shorter than she would be in comparison to her peers makes less of a difference when she's in a chair and interacting at that level. She will still mature at the same level as her classmates. If you look at her face, it will continue to age appropriately. We haven't attempted to change her outward appearance. What we've done is made her shorter than she ultimately would be.[5]

Noted 'ethics expert' Peter Singer was reported in the *New York Times* as saying:

What matters in Ashley's life is that she should not suffer, and that she should be able to enjoy whatever she is capable of enjoying. . . . Lofty talk about human dignity should not stand in the way of children like her getting the treatment that is best both for them and their families.[6]

However, Arthur Caplan, an equally renowned 'ethics expert', sees the case as I do:

I understand the parents' logic. And I can even understand how a medical team might come to agree that a person who cannot move will have a better life small than big. But I think the Peter Pan option is morally wrong. . . . True, it may be better if Ashley does not become sexually developed in terms of protecting her from attack. But that can be said of any woman. To surgically remove her breasts is simply to maim her in a way that ought not be done. She needs a safe environment at home and if the day comes, a safe environment in an institution. Lopping off her breasts to keep her safe cannot be the right or the only answer.

The problems Ashley and her parents face are terribly real. But permanently freezing a person into childhood is not the solution.[7]

I see the 'Ashley Therapy' as 'dwarfing'. Caplan calls it 'Peter Pan' medicine. On the other hand Singer thinks our ideals are too 'lofty' and Diekema and his colleagues sincerely believe the intervention was morally justified.

Neither side can be said to be objectively right or wrong. There is no independent 'ethics test' available. There's no science here – it's simply different people expressing different, deeply held, feelings, sentiments and preferences.

Commitment, not objectivity

If not even something as caring and supportive as health work can be said to be objectively moral, are we forced to accept that morality is, in the end, nothing more than opinion?

In the first two editions of *Ethics: The Heart of Health Care* I answered: no, we don't have to accept this conclusion. Health work – at least health work according to the foundations theory of health[8] – simply is moral work. If you adhere to the foundations theory and genuinely strive to enable people then you are demonstrably and certainly engaged in moral endeavour.

But using terms like 'genuine', 'work for health' and 'moral endeavour' is a poor substitute for strong philosophy and detailed supporting examples. Consequently, in this Third Edition I answer: yes and no. Yes, what one considers to be moral or immoral is a matter of opinion or preference – it is a value judgement. But no, morality is not merely a matter of opinion or preference – rather it is a matter of making a reasoned, sustainable, emotional commitment to a way of living you as an individual feel at ease with.

The problem with standard approaches to ethics is that they play down or ignore emotion in human thinking. Conventional ethics' advice to act according to principles, Codes of Ethics, ethical theory or 'reason' confuses people, particularly when we encounter situations, like Ashley's, that affect us deeply. When this happens we respond instinctively – we usually feel strongly positive or negative – and become highly emotionally engaged. We are often even physically affected – we may flush, our pulse rate may rise and we may feel adrenaline flow.[9] At such times principles, Codes and academic theory are a very long way removed from our decision-making.

Ethics is not primarily about theory, rules, law or 'expert ethical advice'. These aspects may sometimes play a part in people's reflections – but they are not necessary to ethical thinking and more often than not do not enter into our heads when we try to work out what to do in difficult social situations. We draw on other resources, and people who write ethics texts need to recognise this or else continue to produce material irrelevant to people's social experience.

The worst effect conventional ethics writing can have is to make us feel as if we are somehow overreacting, and that all we really need to do is stand back from a situation to think about it calmly. But of course we cannot stand back from situations because we are human beings embedded inexorably in the social realm – we reason and we feel in roughly equal proportion – and we always do so within a web of social, environmental and biological reality. Ultimately ethics is about making an emotional commitment to ways of living and acting – and to make this commitment we have to be open to our feelings and goals; to other people's feelings and goals; to the physical environment and to social contexts we inhabit; and we have to think carefully too. All these elements are necessary for anyone to become proficient at ethics.

Consequently, the Third Edition's argument extends the first two editions' key points (see points **3–6**, above and the **Introduction to the Second Edition**), rejects its previous wishful thinking about ethical certainty, and tries (particularly in the Rational Fields section overleaf) to show that both reason and emotion are an essential part of ethical reflection.

In a nutshell

The Third Edition argues:

- There is no objective morality.
- People are free to decide what their moral outlooks are, whatever they are, even if other people find their views morally disgusting.
- People hold many different moral outlooks, some of which conflict.
- It is impossible to judge between these different outlooks in an unbiased way.

- We are all able to reflect on our moral commitments from time to time and to change them if we see fit, through personal effort and reflection, as we learn through life.
- If you are a health worker then – in your work at least – your moral commitment should be to a theory of health – to a clear idea about the purpose of your work.
- This should be a specific, meaningful commitment. It should include clear ideas about the goals you seek and about what it is right and wrong to do. Ideally, it should also incorporate a way to think things through when situations are ambiguous.
- I cannot prove I am right about ethics and health, but I can try to convince you to share the commitment I find most moral. I recommend the Foundations Theory of health as the best guiding theory for health workers, and the Ethical Grid and the Values Exchange (www.values-exchange.com) as ideal supports for your deliberations.
- A moral commitment is necessarily an emotional commitment. Ethics is a personal activity which involves all aspects of our being. If you think of the world as being composed of masses of interacting rational fields you can begin to appreciate how our lives are formed by a constant interplay between logic, values and instincts, and better understand what ethics really is.
- Once you see the world like this you know why the Ethical Grid is a flexible framework meant to be open to the widest possible personal interpretation.

◆

Rational fields[10]

Ethical judgements are based on people's opinions, however people's opinions are formed by a broad network of historical, familial, environmental and cultural factors that we all experience and partially share in. The religious believer and the atheist obviously see some things differently, and hold some incompatible views, but this does not mean they have completely unconnected outlooks. Nor does it mean they cannot experience, investigate and learn about each other's preferences and realities.

If the message of the first two editions was 'work for health is a moral endeavour', the message of this edition is 'serious work for health means serious exploration of the evidence, serious attention to one's inner life, and serious listening to others'.

Beyond-the-evidence and within-the-evidence

In order to understand this refined message, and to see why we do not need to descend into moral relativism, it is necessary to explore the relationship between evidence and non-evidence.

The inner circle of the figure overleaf (Figure 2) depicts the world of evidence – the world as it is whatever we think of it. The ellipses outside the inner circle depict the different ways we interpret the world of evidence.

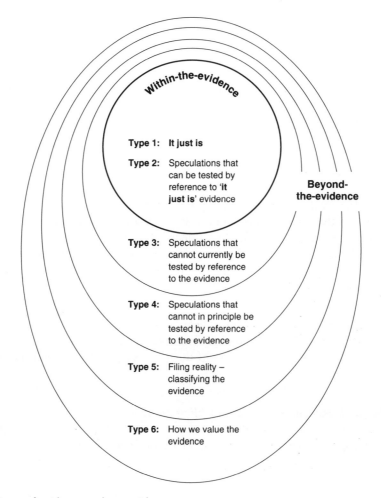

Figure 2 Types of evidence and non-evidence

Within-the-evidence (inner circle)

Type 1: The 'just is' realm

Many events and processes **just are**. For example, it **just is** the case that:

> Breast cancer is the second leading cause of cancer death among North American women. Approximately 1 in 8.2 women will receive a diagnosis of breast cancer during their lifetime, and 1 in 30 will die of the disease.[11] Breast cancer incidence increases with age,[11] and although significant progress has been made in identifying risk factors and genetic markers, more than 50% of cases occur in women without known major predictors.[12–14]

There is no doubting this evidence because it **just is** true.

Type 2: Testable speculations
There are speculations that can be tested by reference to the **just is** evidence. For example, the statements 'screening of women aged 40–49 by mammography can reduce the death rate from breast cancer' and 'life stress is a significant factor in the causation of breast cancer' are both testable by researching the evidence.

Beyond-the-evidence (the ellipses)

Type 3: Speculations that cannot currently be tested
The more we find that the evidence will not yield the explanations we require, the closer we move toward the realm beyond-the-evidence. For example, the speculation that an unknown combination of genetic factors predisposes obese women to a 15% higher chance of contacting breast cancer must remain speculation because we do not yet have sufficient knowledge of genetics to test it out.

Type 4: Speculations that cannot in principle be tested
'It was pre-destined that Amy would experience breast cancer aged 43' and 'Amy's illness is the result of bad karma' are examples of this type, since both speculations are matters of faith not evidence.

Type 5: Human classifications – ways of filing reality
Type 5 is a pervasive and yet under-noticed feature of human life. Not only do we continually make instinctive and intentional beyond-the-evidence decisions to classify evidence into categories, but we must do if we are to make any sense of things at all.

We have to classify the world in order to think about it and act in it. For instance, unless we demarcate desirable behaviour from antisocial behaviour, normal thinking from abnormal thinking, and illness from non-illness – and make countless other daily distinctions – we are powerless to negotiate our social environment.

Type 6: How we value the evidence
Whether we realise it or not, we interpret evidence in accord with our human preferences. And the way we value evidence in turn affects and is affected by our speculations and classifications.

While it might look to us that all our decision-making takes place within the technical rationality ellipse (also called a Spock Bubble[10]), in truth we can't even begin to formulate a logical plan without the influence of the surrounding factors (depicted in the rectangles in Figure 3 – and also in ellipses 3–6 in Figure 2).

Rational fields and their causative influences provide a means of working practically and ethically to improve the social world, using evidence and values in their proper balance.[15]

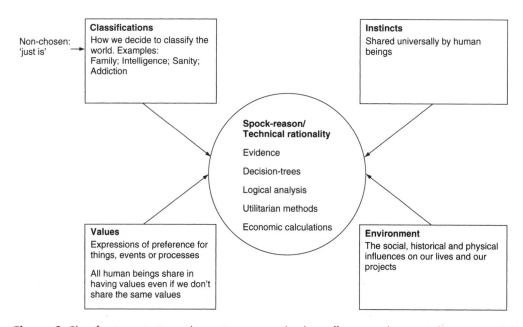

Figure 3 Classifications, instincts, the environment and values affect our selection and interpretation of the evidence

All rational fields have the same basic structure.[16–20] They are formed by any kind of problem-solving behaviour, and can therefore be any size from minuscule to enormous. A rational field is usually created by either an instinct, a value judgement, a behaviour or a plan which generate goals and sub-goals, strategies and sub-strategies, each of which maintain the rational field.

Natural and manufactured rational fields

Natural rational fields

The living world is composed of innumerable rational fields. A plant striving to grow and to propagate is a rational field. A bacterium is a rational field, a cell in a body is a rational field, a gene is a rational field, organs in the human body are rational fields, a developing person is a rational field: anything instinctively purposive is a natural rational field. All these examples have goals and sub-goals, strategies and sub-strategies, each of which maintain their respective rational fields. If new problems emerge, each rational field is likely to expand or adapt in order to try to deal with them. For example, in ideal circumstances a plant will grow and produce many seeds. If there is a drought, if the plant is attacked by insects or if there is excessive wind, then if it can the plant will adapt its goals and strategies accordingly (perhaps it will make only one fruit instead of many, or perhaps it will produce special chemicals to repel further insect attack, or perhaps it will grow extra roots as an anchor). This adaptive behaviour is true of any natural, goal-directed system.[20]

This **just is** the way the world is – natural rational fields exist within-the-evidence.

Because of the world's interconnectedness no natural rational field is wholly independent. However, any rational field must have at least one distinct purpose and strategy by which to pursue that purpose.

Manufactured rational fields

Manufactured rational fields are different from natural ones. They are also goal-directed (they must be to be rational fields) but they tend to be more erratic and unstable than natural rational fields, since they are brought into being by human beyond-the-evidence assumptions and decisions.

Manufactured rational fields are formed and sustained by our classifications of reality (Type 5), our values (Type 6) and our instincts (Figure 3). Manufactured rational fields can be as small as a plan to read a book with a glass of wine, and as big as it is possible for any human institution to be. Conventional health services are manufactured rational fields, a major software company is a manufactured rational field, a major software company marketing department is a manufactured rational field, and so are psychiatry, nursing, a badminton club and the law of the land – every system designed by humans to achieve a purpose is a manufactured rational field.

Once we can recognise manufactured rational fields for what they are we can take control over them. Once we know what we are dealing with we do not have to fall into rational fields that suit other people more than they suit us, and we do not have to follow particular goal-directed paths in the false belief that these paths are all there is.

An example of a simple manufactured rational field

A traveller unexpectedly lost in a foreign city, unable to speak or read the native language, must define a goal and devise ways to achieve it if she wants to regain her bearings. She might think: I don't want to be lost (a value judgement or instinct which defines the ellipses perimeter – Figure 3); if I find the central railway station I will probably find a map (two related goals); if I draw a picture of a train with a question mark and show it around I may get directions to the station (two related strategies); first I need to find some paper (sub-goal), and so on. By doing these things she creates a small rational field. As she formulates and tries strategies to achieve her goal the field expands. As soon as she is successful, the rational field dissipates (the bubble bursts).

An example of a complex manufactured rational field

Large organisations such as hospitals and commercial companies create and perpetuate vast and complex rational fields. Just like the traveller's field, these larger fields are initially created by classifications and value judgements or instincts (we must treat disease, we must improve our brand recognition) which generate further goals and sub-goals, strategies and sub-strategies, each of which contributes to the rational field's evolution.

To describe the relationships between the goals, strategies and means of an organisation the size of BP is a virtually impossible task – even the most determinedly extensive depiction of BP's rational field would be an oversimplification. Fortunately the exact details don't matter – it is the basic *structure* and *formation* of rational fields that needs to be understood. If you know this then you can assess any manufactured rational field for coherence and value base, and can also manufacture a rational field according to your own classifications and values.

The rational field template

Logic, evidence and our perceptions are inextricably entwined – if we display the elements using the rational field template then we can understand and assess this relationship in order to make informed and practical decisions.

All rational fields, whether natural or manufactured, can be depicted like this (Figure 4):

A plant's instinctive rational field response to an attack by an insect might be illustrated like this:

Figure 5 is a natural rational field. Its means are well-related to its goals, and its goals are compatible. Some loss of optimal normal functioning is tolerated in order to achieve goal 2.

A major software company's **manufactured** rational field response to the surprise emergence of revolutionary software from a rival company might (again very crudely) be illustrated as in Figure 6.

In Figure 6 the company's decision is to adopt Strategy Two, to try to prevent the rival launching its product, in order to give the major software company time to increase its own research and development efforts. It is very easy to see how decision trees and other cost–benefit based assessments might be built into the rational field.

It is not suggested that the solution offered in Figure 6 is what the major software company would actually do. Rather, it is an illustrative response, meant only to portray the idea of a manufactured rational field.

At this stage, the main points to note about rational fields are:

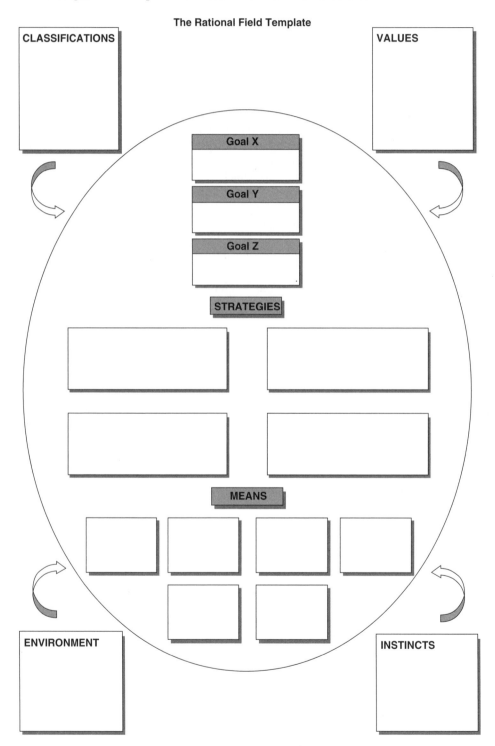

Figure 4 The basic rational field template

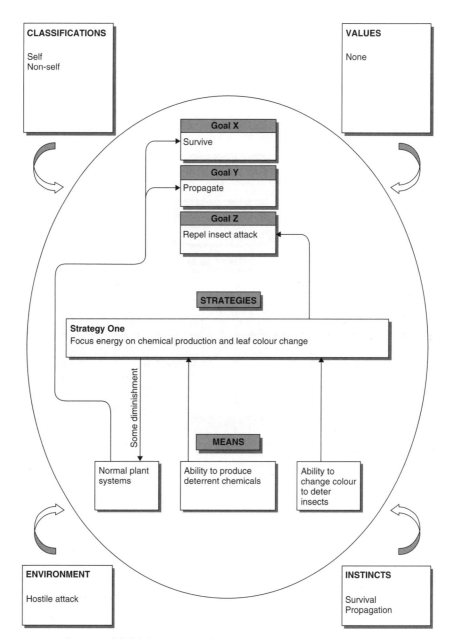

Figure 5 A simple rational field depicting a plant's response to insect attack

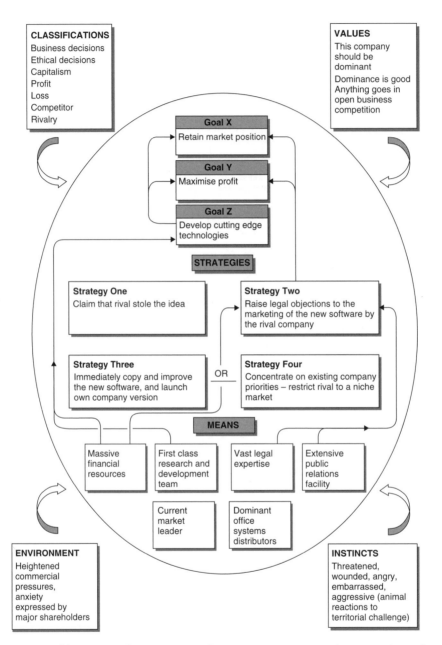

Figure 6 A possible response from a major software company to a rival company's revolutionary software

1 Even simply expressed, the rational field template is useful because it enables decision-makers to state their most important goals, crudely to check whether these goals are compatible with each other, to define and lay out different strategies, to see how these impact on the goals (some may fit with one goal but not another, for example), to state the primary means for achieving any goals, and to assess whether the means, strategies and goals are coherent and efficient (standard matters of technical rationality).

2 More importantly, it is possible, by using the rational field template, to see how a rational field is formed from beyond-the-evidence. In addition to a simple internal field made up of means, strategies and goals, the rational field template shows four boxes – one for instincts, one for classifications, one for values and one for environment – that explain why the internal goals and strategies have been selected. Instincts, classifications, values and the environment shape the rational field entirely – they form its walls. Usually, in our social affairs, we tend not to notice or we play down these elements (as in typical ethics texts and courses). But it is only by properly understanding them that we can understand ourselves and our plans.

Evidence is never decisive when human beings make decisions. Trace any judgement back to its roots and you will, without exception, find a value of some kind. It might, for example, be decided that 'we' (i.e. law abiding, non-terrorist citizens) obviously need increasingly better security procedures at international airports. Yet in fact this is not an obvious decision – rather it is a judgement based on values (our preference to feel as secure as possible inside airports), human classification (there are 'terrorists' and there are 'the rest of us') and instinct (most people are naturally afraid of hidden threats).

We are unlikely to change our preference for safety, and our instincts **just are**. It is, however, open to us to alter our classification of others (for example, from 'terrorists' to 'neighbours') and to do so on the ground of an alternative value – perhaps the Christian edict that we should love our neighbours as ourselves. If we were to start from this latter value base we would come up with a very different strategy from one derived from the atavistic reaction that we should 'take revenge on evil terrorists everywhere'.

Once we have decided we need better security at international airports, subsidiary questions follow – for example, 'How shall we meet our perceived need?' These questions also require values if they are to be answered. Should we, for instance, work out what sort of security to provide according to cost, aesthetics, or civil liberties? Should we invest more in armed police or more in improved surveillance technology? Should we make a truce with our enemies? Or should we simply decide according to 'what works best'? (Of course, there is no escape: 'what works best' depends on what is meant by 'best', and what counts as 'best' depends on human preferences. Value judgements are everywhere.)

Rational fields and the 'Ashley Therapy'

My personal values base tells me that Ashley's parents were morally wrong to do what they did. But it seems there is nothing I can possibly say that will convince them to adopt my moral outlook. And, equally, nothing they can say to me to convince me that they are right.

Apparently it is stalemate: but by using rational fields – and by understanding that morality is not about objective truth but commitment – it becomes at least a little easier to engage in respectful conversation about what best to do.

This would not happen using the traditional ethics routes introduced in **Chapter Six** of this book – we'd quickly end up disagreeing about what 'utility' means; or what our duties are; or about how to interpret principles, or some mess of all three. Yet – if both parties could sit down and complete a **general foundations rational field template** (shown in Figure 7) it could be a revelation.

Here's how I might possibly interpret the template, were I Ashley's father (Figure 8).

Though questions of evidence can be decided by scientific testing of some kind, it is impossible to decide impartially which of the two rational fields (Figure 9) – mine, or what I have presented hypothetically as Ashley's parents' possible field – is more ethical, for there is no objective viewpoint. The only way to judge between these alternative ways of looking at things is to view the rational field from a further rational field.

This may look like an infinite regress – an endless spiral to nowhere. It may look like we are all locked into our own small-minded prejudices. But we are not because we can see rational fields other than our own so long as we have the insight and courage to look.

The beauty of rational fields is that it is possible to expose them – as they are displayed below – to *mutual* scrutiny:

This is what I think. These are the primary factors I believe are influencing my logic. Here is my logic. Here is your logic. Here are the primary factors you say are influencing your logic. Here is what you think. Is this really what you think? Is this really what I think? Is this how you feel? Is this how I feel?

This is the way to experience difference and sameness at once. At the very least, everyone can see that we all use rational fields.

Similarities between the hypothetical rational fields for Ashley's parents and my own 'were I her father'

1 The way I have expressed both fields, the means are identical.
2 Two of the strategies are essentially identical – albeit used for different goals.
3 The environment is – or would be – largely the same (assuming I had gone to the same doctors for medical advice about what to do for Ashley for the best).
4 Some of the instincts are the same.
5 Two out of three goals are the same.

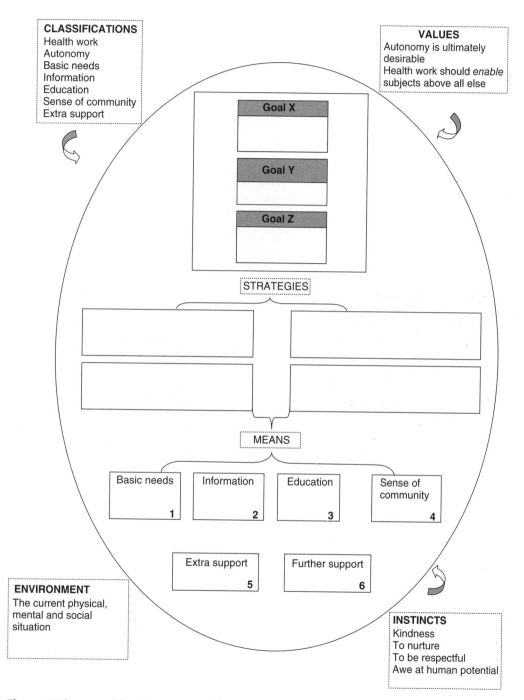

Figure 7 The general foundations rational field template

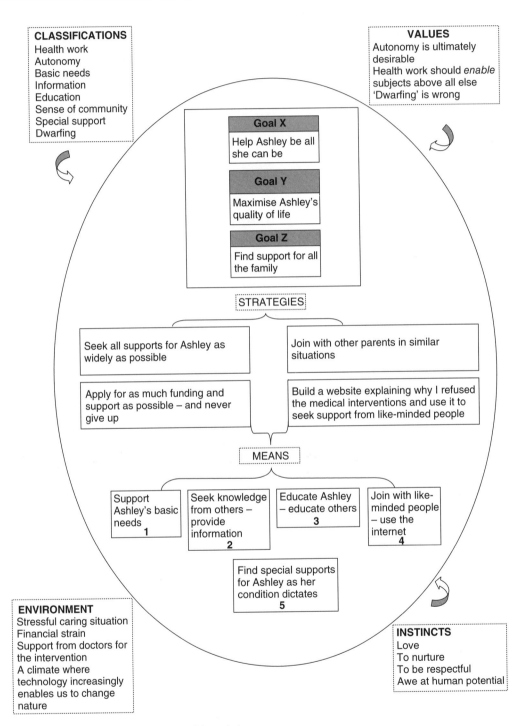

Figure 8 My rational field were I Ashley's father

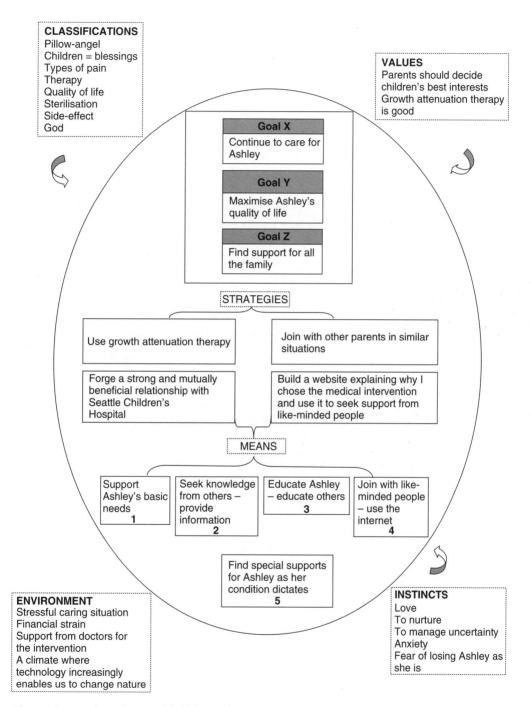

CLASSIFICATIONS
Pillow-angel
Children = blessings
Types of pain
Therapy
Quality of life
Sterilisation
Side-effect
God

VALUES
Parents should decide
children's best interests
Growth attenuation therapy
is good

Goal X
Continue to care for
Ashley

Goal Y
Maximise Ashley's
quality of life

Goal Z
Find support for all
the family

STRATEGIES

Use growth attenuation therapy

Join with other parents in similar
situations

Forge a strong and mutually
beneficial relationship with
Seattle Children's
Hospital

Build a website explaining why I
chose the medical intervention
and use it to seek support from
like-minded people

MEANS

Support
Ashley's basic
needs
1

Seek knowledge
from others –
provide
information
2

Educate Ashley
– educate others
3

Join with like-
minded people
– use the
internet
4

Find special supports
for Ashley as her
condition dictates
5

ENVIRONMENT
Stressful caring situation
Financial strain
Support from doctors for
the intervention
A climate where
technology increasingly
enables us to change nature

INSTINCTS
Love
To nurture
To manage uncertainty
Anxiety
Fear of losing Ashley as
she is

Figure 9 Hypothetical rational field for Ashley's parents based on comments on the Ashley website

Differences between the hypothetical rational fields for Ashley's parents and my own 'were I her father'

1 Goal X
2 (Arguably) awe at human potential
3 Two strategies
4 Key classifications
5 Values

In this case it is especially rewarding to look at the differences between the classifications.

My classifications are included in some books[1,8,10,15] and have been developed over several years – they also are a basic part of my personal Ethics B (see the **Introduction to the Second Edition**).

The hypothetical rational field for Ashley's parents and the classifications it contains have been based on comments appearing on their website. It shows, as it would for everyone else's, a possible rational field (the middle, logical bit) which is inspired by the way they see the world. And it is by exploring what these classifications mean, and what their implications are, that we might find ways of coming together. Like my classification of health, the parents' classifications would be central to the formation of their rational field.

Pillow-angel

They say on their website (reproduced with permission from http://ashleytreatment. spaces.live.com/blog):

> We're often huddled around her holding her hand, thus sensing a powerful connection with her pure, innocent and angelic spirit.[4]

They think they have an angel on their pillow – but it would be equally possible to classify Ashley in any number of other ways: as mentally defective; as a burden; as profoundly learning disabled; as a human being; as a unique person (not an angel). Just like mine, their classifications of Ashley are completely values based.

Children = blessings

This classification, with its implications of possession and ownership, implies that Ashley is their personal blessing, something God has given them. But look how Ashley changes if you apply my classifications – she changes from a 'pillow angel' and their 'blessing' into a unique individual with goals and desires of her own. Perhaps there is room to talk about this?

Types of pain

The parents talk about certain sorts of pain: skin sores, uterine cancer, menstrual discomfort and pneumonia, for example. But there are contrary pains too – for example, the pain of the surgery. And they avoid talking about the potential pain of being so short; of being perceived by others as freakish; by Ashley not having breasts as a woman; of how she will survive in this moulded condition when she is much older and when the parents have died and can no longer care for and protect her.

Therapy

The parents and doctors call their actions therapy – yet they can also and equally be seen as mutilation and manipulation.

Quality of life

This is a subjective term.

Sterilisation

On their website the parents say:

> There was one legal issue that we needed to investigate related to 'sterilization' of a disabled person. Upon consultation with a lawyer specializing in disability law, we found out that the law does not apply to Ashley's case due to the severity of her disability, which makes voluntary reproduction impossible. The law is intended to protect women with mild disability who might chose to become pregnant at some future point, and should have the right to do so.[4]

They enclose the word 'sterilization' in quotes – since they appreciate the importance of classification. Pillow-angels can't be sterilised. They can be doctored to keep them as pillow angels but they cannot be sterilised because this classification does not fit with the parents' values base.

Side-effect

Equally obviously the parents' choice of classification springs directly from their values base when they talk of 'side-effect':

> Furthermore, 'sterilization' is a side effect of the 'Ashley Treatment' and not its intent.[4]

To call something a side-effect is to classify it as less important than the 'real' or 'intended' effects, but there is nothing whatsoever objective about doing this. They are just effects of interventions – how we choose to rank the importance of these effects depends upon our values.

God

Ashley's parents say:

> Some question how God might view this treatment. The God we know wants Ashley to have a good quality of life and wants her parents to be diligent about using every resource at their

disposal (including the brains that He endowed them with) to maximize her quality of life. Knowingly allowing avoidable suffering for a helpless and disabled child can't be a good thing in the eyes of God. Furthermore, the God we know wants us to actively share our experience and learning with the rest of the world to help all 'Pillow Angels' and other special need children in reaping the benefits of the 'Ashley Treatment'.[4]

Clearly this is their view of God; they classify the God they want, regardless of the illogic that their God created a helpless and disabled child in the first place.

If we lay out the competing rational fields, side by side, it becomes very much harder simply to dismiss any of them as simply wrong or immoral. Using rational fields gives us the scope for mutual, trusting exploration – happily this is also the effect of the Values Exchange explained in **Chapter Eleven**.

The truth about relativism

We are now in a much better position to understand how different people come to see the world so differently from one another, and therefore we are in a much better position to understand what is required to be ethical.

Taking a step back to transcend relativism

I and Ashley's parents, like everyone else, continually create billions of natural and manufactured rational fields of varying degrees of compatibility and incompatibility. But we do not have to be trapped within specific rational fields. So long as we are aware (even dimly aware) of the processes which generate any given field we can rise above it to consider what created it. And as we do that we can – just possibly – begin to see things the way people who have very different rational fields from us see things.

If I take the basic Figure 3 above it may look as if we are trapped. It may seem that we are corralled – forced into restricted rational fields by the surrounding causes (just as psychiatrists, soldiers, politicians and lawyers are forced more and more to inhabit specific technical fields – buying into their classifications and values in order to be allowed to be psychiatrists or soldiers at all).

But Figure 3 is merely illustrative. To see the real picture you need to imagine billions of mini-rational fields (the ellipses in Figure 10), each with its surrounding causes (note: it also makes sense to see the whole figure as a rational field, not just the logical part).

At any time any human being will have innumerable rational fields (I need to finish this section by 12.15 p.m. in order to go swimming, I need to lower the volume of my rock music so I can think clearly, I need to drink my cup of tea, I need to stretch my arms, I need to think about rationality, my body is breathing, I am perspiring, my heart is beating, haemoglobin is pumping around my body, I can hear birds singing in the bush outside, etc. etc. etc., almost *ad infinitum . . .*).

We know from personal experience that we can transcend our own rational fields to see them simultaneously, and quite often we can understand their causes. Think about your own rational fields right now. As you do so you create yet another rational field (one with the goal of reviewing your current rational fields and their causes, created by your understanding the classification 'rational field' and your valuing giving my argument

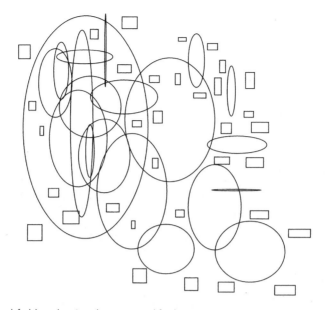

Figure 10 Rational field reality (vastly over-simplified)

a reasonable hearing). This additional rational field gives us a mind's eye view of the sea of rational fields which constitute ourselves and our projects.

We never have to be trapped within any manufactured rational field, so long as we can take this step back. We can even see this mind's eye rational field as we think about it, so creating a further rational field, and so on.

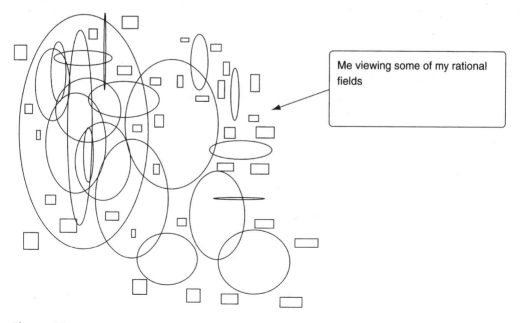

Me viewing some of my rational fields

Figure 11

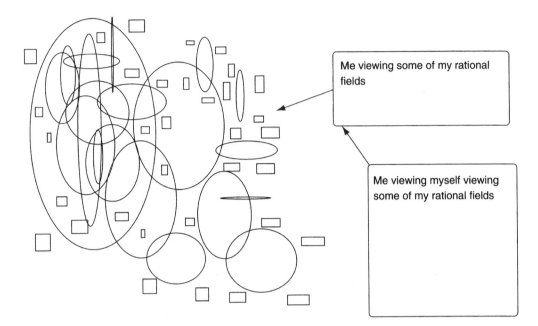

Figure 12

We can sensibly extend this to include ourselves viewing rational fields that are not our own.

Figure 13

Me viewing rational fields which are not my own

Me viewing me viewing rational fields which are not my own

Another person viewing me viewing rational fields which are not my own

Figure 14

From an academic point of view this may look absurd – an infinite regress (like oneself thinking about oneself thinking about oneself thinking about oneself thinking . . .). But in reality this **just is** what happens (in reality I just can't think about myself thinking about myself thinking *ad infinitum*).

Somehow we have to distance ourselves – even if only a little. Perpetual reflection and reviewing, appreciating the proper balance between reason and passion is a far more optimistic standpoint than accepting absolute relativism. It raises the prospect of knowledge, understanding and conversation and is exactly the intent of the Values Exchange explained in **Chapter Eleven**.

Trying to understand the interplay between rational fields is something every one of us can attempt. Everyone – Muslim or Christian, man or woman, black or white – can understand the concept of rational fields and every competent person has a grasp of logic and reason at some level. We share in this understanding because we are human beings – and this is the great hope for us. See values in their proper relationship with logic and

Figure 15 Using the mind's eye to reflect on and consider changing the rational fields that one can change

there is real hope for honesty, openness and insight (though never full agreement) rather than covertness, hostility and blindness to other people's points of view.

By standing back I can review my classifications, instincts, values, environment and logic whenever I want to. I have the potential to decide if the rational field I am currently using is TRULY the rational field I want to be using. Isn't this what we should all be doing?

If I am right about rational fields, the world is a great mass of bubbles – billions and trillions of bubbles – bubbles everywhere, each of which is a rational field, overlapping in ways that cannot be pictured by us.

The big picture is like a many-dimensional snowstorm. We would need to be able to think in other dimensions to see rational fields properly. Whereas snowflakes exist in discreet places, rational fields can be in many places at once, and can overlap in multiple ways with multiple other rational fields, in an incredible complexity. For example, one person's rational field to go to a memorial service is not separate from others within him (his memories, his fears, his hopes, his sense of self). It connects to his other rational fields and other people's rational fields in all sorts of ways – so the whole picture cannot be seen at once – it can be depicted only if we artificially abstract individuals and fields from the great overall mass.

As far as this idea can be explained, rational fields constantly overlap, merge, collide, burst, pop into existence and pop out of existence – in a sub-atomic world of overwhelming complexity.

But if this is the reality then ethical thinking must accept and reflect it.

Summary: everyone is an ethics practitioner

We swim in a sea of ethical processes in which there are no objectively right answers to be found – no matter how clever the ethical theory, no matter how many 'ethics experts' tell us we should agree with their 'ethical truths', and no matter how obvious current answers may seem. There is no ethical touchstone to discover in this swirling ocean. All we have at bottom is ourselves and what we choose to commit to – as far as circumstances permit it is we and only we who decide where and how to swim in the ethical sea.

To 'be ethical' as a health worker – or as anything else in human life – one has to take account of BOTH evidence and logic AND the influence of history, the environment, human instincts, the way we have decided to classify the world and – ultimately – our values.

Values, evidence and reasoning in balance is the key. Not ethical theory, Codes, committees or 'ethics experts' – sometimes these can help us achieve a balanced view, but technical ethics on its own is definitely not the answer.

We are volatile, emotional creatures who – when we create plans – create rational fields. To practice with ethical heart we need to recognise these fields.

Despite many changes from the First Edition, the abiding message of *Ethics: The Heart of Health Care* remains the same.

First, ethics is everywhere – in other words human life has constant and continual ethical content – we just don't notice it because we get used to conventional solutions. Even so, we frequently encounter ethical issues (where we have to decide how to behave when there are no rules to help us) and we deal with them without recourse to ethics text books and ethics experts. So, as we go through life, we are each of us, automatically, ethics practitioners.

However, as in any life practice, it is possible to improve. *Ethics: The Heart of Health Care* was always intended as a practical guide to making better ethical decisions, and it still is. Whether you use the Rings of Uncertainty, the Ethical Grid or the Values Exchange (www. values-exchange.com) you will be challenged to picture yourself and your situation in a personal and social reality – not divorced into the pseudo-intellectual realm preferred by most 'ethics experts'. Ethics is the heart of health care because it requires the heart to commit to a personal, vulnerable, reflective position about what matters most in life. You won't find ethics in the rule books.

David Seedhouse
Auckland, New Zealand
December 2007

Introduction to the Second Edition

There ought to be two reasons why this book has been successful but I suspect there is only one. *Ethics: The Heart of Health Care* has been studied for a decade because it offers down-to-earth guidance to those who want to analyse ethical problems for themselves.

Its practical elements were devised partly to meet a personal need. Between 1984 and 1987 (when the book was completed) I was a junior researcher in a department of health studies, and later a lecturer in a post shared between departments of general practice and community health. My degrees were in philosophy, and I had a reputation for asking apparently facetious questions: what is health? what is special about your work as a nurse? what are the limits of your professional role, doctor? Why I was employed in these institutions was not – I confess – immediately obvious to all my colleagues. However, interest in ethics was escalating in the mid-1980s health world (for reasons I did not then properly comprehend) and I became known as the local 'ethics person'.

Teaching ethics

I quickly learnt that in academic institutions burgeoning interest in a subject does not necessarily imply a similar level of resource with which to study it – in fact there is sometimes a strikingly inverse relationship between these factors. There was usually no room for ethics in official curricula, and the meetings I was asked to lead were squeezed into lunchtime slots or stitched into other courses (they still are sometimes). All of which meant that I typically had no more than 50 minutes to explain ethics from scratch to groups of strangers.

My earliest attempts suffered not only from lack of time, but also from my ignorance of the practicalities of orthodox health care. A novice of health service reality
teaching newcomers to ethics over a snatched sandwich was unlikely to be an overwhelming success. I would try to explain different theories in moral philosophy while
my students would patiently introduce me to such essentials as medical/nursing hierarchies, 'not for resuscitation' notes and the irrationality of health service decision-
making. On the best days both parties would learn a little from the other, but we
never managed to get beyond the basics, and were rarely able to begin analysis
proper.

Despite these repeated stumbles, it became clear both that I would continue to receive
invitations to teach ethics to groups of health workers, and that I was unlikely to be
allowed more time to do it. I needed something more if I was to continue to accept these
offers – I needed a framework which would enable me to present complex ideas rapidly
and accessibly, and which would also ensure that realistic solutions could be offered to
the students' endless practical problems.

This was asking a lot, but I did have assets on which to build. I had already developed
a theory about the importance and purpose of health work, I had a brilliant friend and
colleague to talk to, I was willing to make a compromise between the purity of philosophy
and the murkiness of practice, and I very much wanted to be useful. These attributes
combined to produce the Ethical Grid.

Spider's web or ethical template?

If I had not been able to discuss health care ethics and how to teach it with Alan Cribb
I would not have come up with the Ethical Grid. I remember a conversation with Alan
over a beer (several in my case) in a Manchester pub. We were discussing the pervasiveness of ethics in health care, and bemoaning the perception that ethics is only of periph-
eral concern for health workers. I think I may have asked Alan to tell me the main
components of health ethics, as he saw them.

I cannot recall the details, but I was struck by the image he proposed. He said – I
think – that it is an error to think of key or organising principles in ethics. Rather one
should conceive of ethics as a 'spider's web' in which each idea is connected to all other
ideas by all manner of routes, and where each is partly responsible for the strength of
the web as a whole. In different circumstances different parts of the web may be more
useful than others, but all may be needed – a fly can land on any part of a spider's web,
after all.

But Alan's idea was not that ethics is a way to 'trap a problem'. He was explaining
that wherever one starts in a deliberation (whether one considers rights, duties, consequences, virtues or principles), if the deliberation is done thoroughly one will either
have to visit the other areas at some point, or will receive implicit support from them.
If you are a doctor anxious to know whether you have a duty to tell your patient's
partner something she wants kept secret, you must reflect on matters beyond duty
(what will happen if I do this rather than that? who will benefit? who will suffer?
who is entitled to know what? is negotiation possible? is there a way to avoid confrontation?). Good ethics is comprehensive deliberation about the pros and cons of
action.

Alan had expressed a powerful insight into the nature of ethics, and I thought for a while that this might be the answer to my teaching problem. However, what was enlightening to me – a trained philosopher – proved too complicated for the inexperienced audience I was trying to teach: I needed something equally philosophically illuminating, but simpler to apply.

Somehow the 'ethical web' changed, in my imagination, into a much less beautiful piece of engineering. I pushed, pulled and chopped it until it became a group of simple, transparent squares, on each of which a key ethical word or notion was inscribed. My idea was that this 'ethical template' (as I then saw it) could be 'placed over' a situation by the reasoner and – dependent upon which part of the template was superimposed – could bring a solution into focus.

This was not a good idea, not least because it was too rigid – the antithesis of the understanding of ethics Alan and I shared. For example, I had in mind something like this:

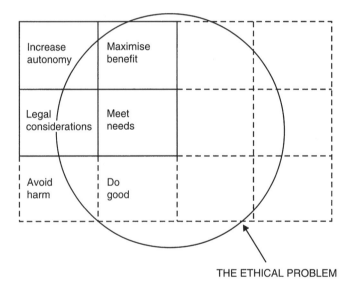

THE ETHICAL PROBLEM

Figure 16 The ethical template superimposed over an ethical problem

However, the association of boxes was not only arbitrary but also fixed. Most problems would require boxes from various parts of the template – a box from here, another from there – so making superimposition impossible.

My next proposal – almost as inadequate as the static template – was to design the teaching tool to resemble a game in which the player moves squares in a fixed frame. One square is missing and the challenge is to juggle squares round this space until the required arrangement is produced (in some versions of the commercial game the aim is to arrange numbers or letters in the right order). I envisaged the ethical reasoner moving transparent pieces until he hit on the right combination to 'place over' the ethical problem, like this (Figure 17):

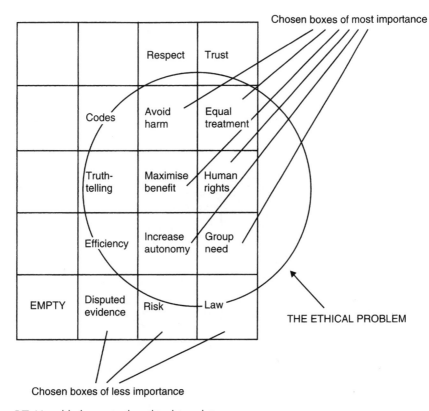

Figure 17 Movable boxes in the ethical template

Not only was this too cumbersome, it also had the effect of focusing the reasoner's attention more on the 'game' and how to move the squares around than on the ethical problem itself. I had to find a way to include all the essential squares and words within a clearly defined structure (to help students grasp immediately that ethical analysis can be kept within bounds), but with flexibility of use and interpretation. And thus it was that I sat down with the template – boxes arranged randomly in a square – three coloured felt tip pens, and the determination to make a difference to the education of health workers, to produce the version of the Ethical Grid published in the First Edition.

This (Figure 18) looked too much like a dart-board. So in the printed version I retained the idea of angular movable boxes but removed them from the over-restrictive frame. Instead, I arranged them in four distinct layers (see **Chapter Nine**): black for practicalities, green for outcomes, red for duties and blue for health work purpose. This gave the Grid sufficient rigidity to prevent disorientation amongst new users while permitting considerable fluidity of application.

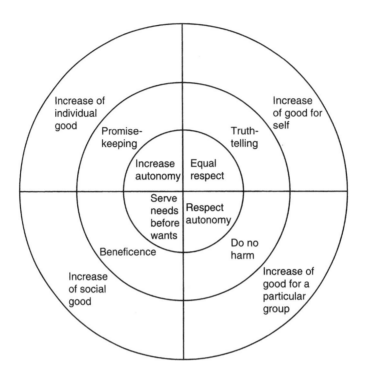

Figure 18 An early version of the Ethical Grid

The secret reason for the book's success

If this had been all there was to my thinking, if *Ethics: The Heart of Health Care* was merely the Ethical Grid plus summaries of ethical theory, and the Grid little more than a loose collection of coloured labels, I would not have published. If I had intended the book to be 'gimmicky' or 'ethics by rote' as some unperceptive reviewers seemed to think, I would have been wasting my time writing it. Worse, I would have been deceiving readers about the nature of health care ethics, when my real purpose was to facilitate improved deliberation about pressing practical problems.

Because the book is so accessible and uncomplicated I fear that both general reader and scholarly critic alike have tended to overlook just *why* it is so clear. The book looks so straightforward it is hard to imagine there is more to it than meets the eye. But there is. It is not written in an elaborate 'academic style' – non-academics can understand it – and it is simple in the most positive sense of the word. But it is also theoretically rich. If it were not underpinned by a strong theory it would not be so easy to read, and I have no doubt it would have suffered the fate of countless more scholarly ethics books, consigned to one small print run and then isolation on some obscure library shelf.

In this new introduction, permit me the luxury of outlining the hidden reason for the book's success. Let me explain first that *Ethics: The Heart of Health Care* is Part

II of a still growing series – the sequel to an earlier book and one part of a now sizable body of work. Allow me to add a little more theory – let me explain the moral importance of *committing* to a theory of health. Let me briefly summarise what some may have missed in the First Edition. And finally let me tell a frightening personal story which renewed my ethical fervour, and brought home just how much further there is to go.

Foundations two

In 1985, 2 years before I wrote *Ethics: The Heart of Health Care*, I completed the manuscript for my first book, *Health: The Foundations for Achievement*.[8] This project sought to discover a theoretically and practically defensible answer to the question: what is health? Various theories of health were surveyed and discussed, and each was found wanting in important respects. However, my analysis revealed that all theories of health (certainly all the theories I came across) and all practical work done in health's name, stated or implied that work for health is done in order to remove actual or perceived obstacles to the achievement of biological or chosen human potentials. Health work, in other words, aims to liberate fulfilling human potential by the prevention, elimination or alleviation of impediment: the nurse offering a careful explanation to an excitable patient, the general practitioner sending blood samples to a lab for testing, the psychiatrist seeking the best combination of medications to reduce a patient's mental turmoil, the public health specialist investigating the cause of an outbreak of food poisoning – each of these is doing what is professionally expected and each is working to tackle obstacles to desirable and/or biologically normal human growth.

In *Foundations* I developed this observation into a theory of health intended to display the theoretical limits to health work, and so help practitioners work out more exactly what their role is – to help them decide when they should begin to intervene, which interventions are legitimate and which not, and when they must withdraw from situations. As I developed this theory I was at the same time developing an account of the ethics of health work, though I did not realise it at the time.

Health: The Foundations for Achievement does not mention ethics. Though it may be hard to believe, I was so taken up with conceptual analysis I was oblivious to the work's ethical content. I wanted to find out the meaning of health and to show that knowing this could improve practice. It was only later, as I taught my work to a nursing class and gave ethics sessions to other groups, that I slowly put two and two together. I came to understand that there is not one compartment labelled 'the theory of health' and another labelled 'health care ethics', but that it is impossible to think deeply about health without also thinking deeply about morality – and vice versa.

Most books on health, medical and nursing ethics do not appreciate this connection. Instead, their authors take commonly held ethical principles and apply them to health care contexts.[21-23] They have not been developed with health care in mind, and can be applied equally to other social situations. It is rare to find much theoretical support for these principles, and even more unusual to come across reasons why these and not other principles should be brought to bear on health care situations. Unlike *Ethics: The Heart of Health Care* these books tack ethics on to health care. This book, by contrast, is rooted in an understanding of the nature of health (taken from *Foundations*) and develops its ethical argument (and the Ethical Grid) out of this.

The slogan 'work for health is a moral endeavour' is not a throwaway line but meant to announce that there are striking commonalities between what it means to work for health and what it means to be engaged in practical moral deliberation. 'Work for health' is a morally special activity, its purposes more humane and noble than most other human enterprises (including commercial activity, the system of adversarial criminal law and pure mathematics, to give just three examples).

Note too that 'work for health' does not mean only traditional health care, such as doctoring and nursing. These activities can be work for health but are not necessarily so. The terms 'health care' and 'health service' are sometimes used in this text to mean 'medical care' and 'medical service', but it should be remembered that this is not an automatic conjunction. If medical services are not carried out in line with the Foundations Theory of health then they are not health work (in the Foundations sense).

Work for health requires moral commitment

It may be helpful to expand on this point. The body of the book argues that there are no moral standards beyond the human world. This means that no-one is morally obliged to act in any particular way – if you want to behave selfishly no 'moral court' will ever punish you. However, since all social behaviours take place in the moral realm, we continually have a golden opportunity to commit to moral ways of life – if we choose. Those who genuinely wish to work for health must make a knowing commitment to achieving health goals – and this requires commitment to a theory of health. As she commits, the health worker pledges simultaneously to a powerful set of moral obligations – a commitment all the more emphatic because it is voluntary.

If ethics means anything then:

1 Actions, made by competent human beings, which have relevance for other human beings, inescapably have ethical content because they have the potential to affect others for better or worse; and
2 All competent human beings have the capacity to recognise this.

Ethical A and Ethical B

Points 1 and 2 form part of a theory in which there are two forms of the ethical, *ethical A* and *ethical B*, where *ethical A* means *ethical in the sense of having ethical content* and *ethical B* means *ethical in the sense of having a consistent view about what one ought to do in the social world*.

Ethical A is a pervasive phenomenon of (competent) human life. Because we live with others in an ethical realm we constantly encounter ethical situations, whether or not we perceive them as such. Being pleasant, unpleasant (or anything else) to people during a

Saturday morning trip around the supermarket are *ethical A* actions – regardless of intent – because they have the potential to produce different sorts of meaningful consequence.

Not every action is *ethical A*. Those of no relevance to other people lie outside the ethical realm. Idly playing with one's hair, tapping on the desk as one works, reflex responses such as the blink of an eye and so on, are not of ethical interest. Only if they become potentially or actually relevant to others are they *ethical A* actions (if desk-tapping is done in a shared office or if hair twirling becomes an obsession which could interfere with one's relationships, for instance).

Ethical B actions stem from a person's awareness that what she does is socially important. The task for anyone who wishes to be *ethical B* is first to work out what 'being ethical' means, and then to devise the most effective strategy to be it. Since the founding question of ethics is *how should I conduct my life in the presence of other lives?*, the ethical challenge – at any time and in any place – is to work out what *commitment to living* to make. When a desk-tapper who wants to be ethical realises she is being irritating, it is up to her to work out what to do about it. She might decide to stop – or she might reason that she is entitled to continue – but whatever she decides, as she sees that her actions have implications for other people and resolves because of this to behave in a certain way, so she begins to create her *ethics B*.

Health work ethics

Work for health is a certain sort of moral endeavour – a certain sort of *ethical B*. Not only is it generally true that actions made in the social world by competent human beings inevitably have ethical content, but health work – probably more than any other work – *exposes* this *ethical A*. Even something habitually dismissed as trivial – a smile, for instance – is more obviously within the ethical realm in medical work than it is in most other fields of human endeavour: a condescending smile offered to a sensitive and vulnerable patient might be extremely damaging, while a sincere smile of welcome could emancipate. Furthermore, because the *ethical A* is so visible in health work, most health workers find it necessary to commit to some *ethics B* or other. Normally, these *ethics Bs* are either vague (forms of everyday ethics – see p. 17) or based on principles and beliefs derived from sources outside health work (as is the case with almost all positions in medical ethics). Yet it is immeasurably preferable that health workers practise according to a properly thought-out theory about what health work is and why they ought to do it.

Health workers should take as much *command* as they can of the *ethical A* by committing to an *ethics B* based on the foundations theory of work for health. The Ethical Grid is a graphic illustration of this. Its three outer layers are analogous to the *ethical A*, and the blue layer is a simple summary of the *ethics B* I recommend to health workers. It is this *ethics B* that is meant to govern the Ethical Grid.

In Figure 19 the iceberg represents the ethical realm. The matchstick person must live as part of this realm, whether he likes it or not. He must also, if he wishes to *be* ethical, make a commitment to an *ethics B* – to a particular way of living in the social world. To do this properly he needs help. He needs a method to enable him to see the full extent of the iceberg (*ethical A*), and to structure his thinking as he seeks to achieve ethical goals

The choice of tool (Ethics B) – or even *not* to choose a tool at all – is up to the competent person.

At any given time/context only some of Ethical A is at issue (but this is an illusion – we are not looking hard enough)

The person who 'would be ethical' requires a tool (a) to recognise the extent of Ethical A and (b) to act to achieve ethical goals consistently within the Social World/Ethical Realm

Ethics A

The social world *is* the Ethical Realm – it is all we have to stand on

Ethics A

Ethics A

Ethics A

Figure 19 Ethical A and Ethical B illustrated by use of the iceberg

consistently. If he wishes to be a health worker he must commit to an *ethics B* based on a theory of health. He will achieve all these ends if he makes good use of the Ethical Grid.

The book's argument

The particular argument of *Ethics: The Heart of Health Care* also seems to have gone largely unnoticed. It is not clear why (its main steps are spelt out in the unaltered **Preface to the First Edition**). It is worth restating those points that have been most misunderstood, in the hope that the book might yet be seen for what it was meant to be.

A cursory look at **Chapter One** may give the impression that my case was not only naive, but entirely wrong. It may seem that I was merely (and falsely) predicting an imminent paradigm shift – wagering that a version of health care based on my theory of health would shortly supersede health care based on no theory of health. A more careful reading of **Chapter One** will show I was hedging my bets, but I concede that I was hoping that health systems would have moved closer to my ideal, 10 years on. I even expected it in optimistic moments. Yet if anything health systems have become less like Paradigm Y than ever.

Although I did not realise it in 1986–88 (as a young philosopher I was still insulated from the practical world by my training, even though I had begun to work in a health environment) much more influential landmarks were being put in place in the UK, where I was living. I had thought – with woefully little evidence – that the rather romantic list I give on pp. 4–5 of the First Edition amounted to a signpost showing health care's near-future direction. And in this I was wrong, and had missed the writing on the wall in front of me.

Not only had US academics and policy-makers been debating the escalating costs of medical care in that country for two decades, but the Conservative government in the UK was increasingly taking notice of what they had to say. The Tories were rightly concerned that the British NHS, largely run by medics and administrators, was set to absorb ever greater amounts of GDP unless something was done to control spending. Their answer, following a review in 1983, was to introduce 'health management', informed by commercial notions and supported by advice from economists (soon to be commonly known as health economists). In ensuing years this has meant greater emphasis on 'value for money', demonstrable 'outputs', quantification and squeezing as much as possible out of increasingly demoralised staff. Indeed it looks as if Paradigm X has been replaced not by Paradigm Y but by Paradigm Z. It looks as if the old guard, who think health work should be guided by medical priorities, has been overrun by an army of managers who are not particularly concerned what drives the system, so long as its costs are kept in check.

My speculations about the content of Paradigm Y were admittedly idealistic and ill-informed – but then they were meant only as speculations, nothing more. I hoped things were going to get better quickly, but I was to be disappointed. However, speculation aside, I was attempting to offer a solid argument.

1 The crisis that really concerned me was not that which still worries UK and US governments. I was not bothered about transient policy matters. I was interested in the *conceptual* crisis I had discovered as I was researching *Foundations*. I was concerned about the fundamental health care problem, which was that no-one – as far as I could tell – was clear about the point of it. No-one could properly define the purpose of health care, and without this health workers were bound to remain vulnerable to political whim and policy fad.

2 It can be shown that medical services are not necessarily synonymous with health services. Because:

A person's or group's (optimum) state of health is equivalent to the state of the set of conditions which fulfil or enable a person or group to work to fulfil their realistic chosen and biological potentials[24]

not only can work for health be done without reference to medicine and medical priorities but medicine can be practised without it being work for health.

3 Many health workers were dimly aware of 1 and 2 but found themselves frustrated, powerless to do anything to change things for the better. Not only could they not specify what 'better' meant in practice, but they did not possess sufficient theoretical grounding to move toward it.

4 I hoped to offer disaffected health workers the theoretical backing they needed. Since work for health is a moral endeavour it was obvious – to me at least – that if I could help health workers learn how to reason morally (by drawing on a thoughtful combination of moral theory and health philosophy) then their daily practice would provide the impetus for the new era to come, sometime in the future. That is:

> The theories people hold about their everyday work – the subjective theoretical framework in which they operate – can affect their interpretation of what they do. Health workers' understanding of their practice affects both their performance and their attitude towards those for whom they are caring. Since a variety of subjective understandings exist it is surely important to make them overt. . . . By so doing . . . it may then also be possible to shape future developments to correspond with the richest sense of health, by highlighting the most moral understandings of the point of health work . . . it may just be possible to speed the formation of Paradigm Y, to ensure that it emerges with the most enlightened and egalitarian rationale.[25]

Similarly:

> The process of change from one paradigm to another is not definite and predictable. The future must, to an extent, be shaped actively by people. The question is: How is it possible to ensure that the new era of health care that emerges from the period of crisis has the best possible form and content? The route to an answer is opened up by offering health workers a more comprehensive understanding of the nature of ethics. Ethics is the key to the new era of health care. Health workers must know that work for health is a moral endeavour.[26]

5 The Ethical Grid is meant to enable health workers to inject Paradigm Y theory into their everyday practice.

It is impossible to show that answers to practical problems are absolutely ethical. However, it is clear that the deliberate and avoidable *dwarfing* of persons (i.e. most human beings – see **Chapter Six**) is fundamentally immoral, and that the further health workers can distance their practices from dwarfing the more moral their work will be (**note: this position is no longer held in the Third Edition**). Some answers are more ethical than others because they liberate more and better potentials.

The Ethical Grid combines moral theory, health theory and pragmatic context. In addition, the requirement that reasoners use at least one blue box is meant to ensure that practical solutions are inspired by the Foundations theory.

The fact that ethical deliberation can produce varying and even incompatible solutions does not undermine the speculation that by doing ethics a better-shaped health system will emerge. Rather, it is the act of reasoning, critically, honestly and where possible publicly, that will bring about the revolution.

At present too much health care (which is still popularly taken to mean the provision of medical services) is organised hierarchically, and too many health workers are not allowed to think for themselves. Protest is stifled, tradition holds sway, people are able to get away with crass judgements just because they have senior posts or are medically trained, and resources are allocated not through the force of reason but because certain individuals have greater power than others. Of course this is the way of the world. Corruption is part of human life, but there are degrees of it – it is possible to have more or less corruption, to have a more or less principled system, to be more or less honest and to work according to specified theories or not. Things do not have to be the way they are and I maintain, despite the surface evidence, that progress can and will come once enough health workers genuinely and consistently practice ethically, in the sense put forward in this revised text.

It is idealism to imagine that a device such as the Ethical Grid could become a ubiquitous tool of practice – it is too unsettling, too levelling, too challenging to the status quo – but I have seen it used to good effect in many different situations (in critical care, in paediatrics, in nursing, in oncology, in neonatal units) to know that it can work and that health workers feel greater confidence when they use it. Indeed, through using the Grid and studying *Ethics: The Heart of Health Care* thousands of practitioners have discovered that intelligent moral reasoning requires neither formal philosophical training, nor the blind acceptance of dogma. It is not unrealistic to hope that its use will become more widespread still. Perhaps – just perhaps – sufficient health workers will take advantage of it to bring about a tangible shift in the ethos of health care.

The Operation

I was recently vividly reminded why it is so important that Paradigm Y materialises.

I have been developing my position for over 13 years, and had become lulled into thinking that everyone is aware of it. Of course this was a feeble assumption, but nevertheless an easy one to make. Worse still is to assume that not only does everyone now see your point, but they are also acting on it.

The extent to which this is a false belief hit home recently, during an unwanted encounter with an ear, nose and throat surgeon. I relate the tale to show how easily – and how much – harm can be done in ethical ignorance.

A personal experience

For as long as I can recall I had a small, firm, roundish, mobile lump below and slightly forward of my left ear. I didn't worry about it, just fiddled with it occasionally as I shaved (it seemed insignificant and stayed the same size). I mostly forgot it completely. Sometime before Christmas 1996 I noticed it again. It seemed a little bigger, but I couldn't be sure. In any case I couldn't imagine it would be serious. I'm healthy and expect to stay that way, after all.

In early December I went to the GP for a couple of things and mentioned it to her. I could tell, from her immediate distraction, that it might be serious. Instantly I began to feel sick (sick to the stomach and sick that I was in trouble and sickest that this might affect Hilary – my wife – and Charlotte – my daughter). The GP, who seems to have an intuitive understanding of the relationship between ethics and work for health, was straight and to the point:

'You'll need to see an ENT surgeon. You may need an operation. Do you have medical insurance? No? Well it may cost $2000–3000 dollars so we'll try the public system first.'

I stuttered some questions, mostly to establish just how much I should worry:

'I'm 99.9% certain that it isn't cancer. I know what a cancer feels like. I used to work in a hospice.'

'Should I worry about this?'

'No.'

But I did, of course. Dazedly, with the help of Hilary's characteristically perceptive prompting, I wondered. If it's nothing to worry about why do I need to see the ENT surgeon? What exactly is this problem? And later that evening, if it is going to cost $3000 then what will the operation involve?

I managed to put the problem to the back of my mind for at least some of the time and got on as best I could. Just before a brief holiday in Nelson I received an outpatient appointment to Auckland hospital, which made trepidation unavoidable.

I went to the hospital *worried and ignorant.* I emphasise this because – though I'm probably over-anxious – I imagine the great majority of patients in similar situations must feel as I did. And I emphasise it because it must surely be obvious to anyone seeing people in such circumstances that this is how they must be feeling.

After a wait of three-quarters of an hour, in a crowded waiting room, unable to establish how long I would have to wait despite politely asking the receptionist, I was shown into the consulting room by a nurse. Will I get my lump cut out here and now? I thought. I hoped so. I hoped it would be a local anaesthetic and that would be that, but I was forlorn to see a small room, not surgically equipped. I knew already that my worrying would have to go on.

The doctor wasn't there and the nurse was trying to be cheerful – I can't remember what she said but she seemed more nervous than I. She scurried around like a giant mouse. She was about to rush away with my notes when I managed to ask if I could see them. 'Of course', she said, 'these days you have a right to', but she was in so much of a hurry I could read no more than the GP's referral letter which asked for the surgeon's opinion on excision, with the brief history I had given. Thoughtfully my GP had highlighted in pink the sentence: **the patient is senior lecturer in medical ethics at the medical school.**

The surgeon, a conspicuously overweight middle-aged man, breezed in. I stood up – I think he may have held out his hand to introduce himself. He immediately said, 'Where's this lump then?' and felt it as he wished. Almost instantly, or so it seemed to me, he announced, 'You have a benign tumour of the salivary gland' (I didn't know if I was relieved or shocked – I certainly had no idea what this meant). He then directed me toward the examining table and told me to lie down. 'I just want to take a needle biopsy' (I think this was what he said). He didn't ask for permission, and he didn't say there might be any untoward consequences (other than the obvious one of finding out that I had cancer), and I was obedient. It all happened so quickly it is hard to see how I could have objected without causing considerable fuss.

He took his needle and inserted it into my lump. 'This might hurt a bit.' 'Yes', I said. What else do you say? It did hurt a bit – not much, though it hurt more when he wiggled the needle around inside the lump.

As he was doing this he was speaking. Something along these lines:

'So you're a lecturer in ethics are you? Where?'

'At the medical school, across the road.'

'I've not seen you before.'

'I don't see many surgeons.' (This was an attempt at a joke. It went unnoticed.)

'I don't bother with the medical school any more – too socialist for me.'

'Oh no', I said, looking at the nurse out of my left eye, between the needle and the surgeon's arms. She raised her eyebrows. In sympathy, I think.

He squirted the sample between two microscope slides. As he did so he called his registrar in.

'This is Dr blah blah.'

'Hello', I said.

'This patient has blah blah blah.'

What did he say? Before I had time to ask, registrar blah blah had said, 'That's all I need to know', and left the room.

'Thanks, Doc,' I managed.

I was told to sit up and to return to the doctor's desk. I felt shakier than ever.

'You need an operation but there is a risk.'

'OK,' I said. 'What!?' I thought. He showed me what needed to be done. He reached under his left ear and with his right hand made as if to pull back a large flap of skin, just as a cartoon character would remove a mask.

'It is not easy to get at the blah blah. There is a less than 1% chance of damage to the facial nerve. Even if all goes well you'll have a sore left ear and your ear lobe will almost certainly always be numb.'

I couldn't believe this. This wasn't happening.

'What's the worst that can happen?' I was convinced he was going to say 'you'll die.' But he said nothing. Instead he took his finger and pulled the left side of his mouth firmly downwards.

'Oh God', I thought. I knew I wasn't right but I hadn't expected this.

After I told him I hadn't got insurance he put me on the waiting list for the public hospital.

'How long will I wait for?'

'I can't say, you know what a mess the public system is in at the moment – it could be months.'

'Does that matter?'

'No, but the tumour needs to be removed.'

Without meaning to, he then reassured me.

'I won't ask you to wait for the result of the biopsy because I'm virtually certain what it is.'

'When will I know for sure?'

'If you don't hear within a week it is what I think it is.'

At some point – whether before or after this I can't recall – he said, 'Of course, if you went private it could be done much quicker – I have a private practice but I'm not supposed to tell you that here.'

'How much?'

'It could be four and a half thousand.'

'You'd better give me your card.'

'I don't have a card here, but here is the number of my private rooms.'

There were several questions floating in my mind – and I wasn't so thrown I'd forgotten what there were – but he was pointedly waiting to leave so I only managed to put a couple – and these had to be prompts to him.

'So, if I don't have this removed it gets bigger and then that can cause damage?'

'Yes.'

'You think I should get this done?'

'Yes.'

And that was that. I gave my form to the receptionist and reeled out of the ward, unable to think straight, with months of anxiety ahead. I went to my office across the street and called Hilary. She was shocked and upset but had the presence of mind to advise me to call my friend, a retired physician. I told him I had a benign tumour (I hoped) of the salivary gland, and it was from him I learned it was technically a tumour of the parotid gland (though that wasn't what the doctor had said to the registrar, I was sure).

Because I work in a medical school I have access to the library so I read up what I could. I wasn't sure what sort of tumour I had (I discovered there are different sorts of benign parotid tumour) but my friend – on further inquiry – told me he thought it was most likely a mixed-cell tumour. And if so it should come out because though they grow slowly they don't stop – one book had a picture of a man with one the size of a football – and they can suddenly become malignant (which was worse news than ever, but I was so emotionally deadened by now it didn't matter very much).

I told Hilary and we decided to pay for the operation out of our savings. I called the surgeon at his private rooms. After a couple of hours he called back (to his credit he didn't then know that I wanted a private operation). I told him I'd decided to pay and asked when he could do it.

'I'm going on holiday soon but I could do you on Tuesday if you like.' It was Thursday at 4 p.m.

'OK,' I said, my thoughts muffled in a nightmare.

I pulled out of it, and discovered more about parotid tumours from an internet site. This helped explain the doctor's reasoning (my symptoms fitted a pattern typical of a benign tumour). Two days later I had cause to read the site more carefully still.

A cricket test

On the Saturday, aware I was over-anxious about what might happen, I took myself off to the New Zealand vs England cricket Test at Eden Park, Auckland. But though the sunshine baked me I felt bleak, and couldn't concentrate. For no particular reason I decided to move to a seat in the West Stand. As I walked behind the South Stand to get there I was shattered – utterly shattered – to realise that my mouth had filled with blood. I spat it out, oblivious of the spectacle I might make to the other people milling around, but the blood kept coming. Swallowing most of it I went to the Gents for water. I swilled my mouth and saw in the mirror that the lining of my cheek – behind the tumour – seemed to have irregular lines of blood leaking from it.

I felt as if I wasn't there. That's it, I thought. I've had it now. It's cancer and I'm going to die. And at that point I again had the feeling it didn't matter. My – presumably irrational – reaction was if that's it that's it and there's nothing I can do now.

But the blood stopped. It went as quickly as it came. White-faced I bought a diet coke (I had been intending to do this anyway) and walked as if weightless to the West Stand, where I sat in disbelief. No more blood though.

I couldn't sit at the cricket – so I drove to work (a mile away) to phone Hilary. I didn't want to but had to tell her what had happened and we were both upset. I was on the verge of tears, but the bleeding had stopped so I rallied.

I called the doctor's mobile phone but it was switched off. I called his rooms (no answer – it was Saturday). I called the hospital – maybe Dr blah blah the registrar can tell me what it is. I got through to him and explained what had happened. He was quite unconcerned. I think this was actually disinterest but I interpreted it favourably and – as I had done with the surgeon – prompted an answer which had only just occurred to me.

'I assume – I hope – that the blood is something to do with the needle biopsy?'

'Yes', he said casually, 'there are many small ducts which lead to the inside of the mouth. The surgeon must have damaged some, and they must then have clotted. The clot dissolved, that's all. It's nothing to worry about.'

'It's nothing to worry about if you know what it is', I said, with surprising force considering my mental state. But he didn't rise to the bait and said – once I told him I had opted for the private operation.

'I'm sure you'll be alright once my boss has operated. As my grandfather used to say, "a stitch in time saves nine".'

Good grief, I couldn't help thinking, he'll be telling me a spoonful of frigging sugar helps the medicine go down next, but I left it. 'Thanks, Doc,' I said to him for the second time.

I checked on the internet site. Sure enough, here were the risks of needle biopsy, none of which the doctor told me before he took the sample. They are:

Advantages
- Safe, economical, easy to perform, minimal pain
- Often provides a preoperative diagnosis and may obviate the need for surgery in some patients.

Potential problems
- Haemorrhage
- Fistula formation
- Facial nerve injury
- Infection
- Needle tract implantation
- Interpretation difficulties.

Thanks, Doc, I thought.

At the hospital

The ethically barren pattern continued at the hospital, and I confess I found it difficult to cope. It is important to appreciate how I was feeling – a doctor's moral incompetence always has a human context.

I didn't sleep much the night before my operation, partly because I had to be at the hospital by 7 a.m., and I never sleep well if I know I have to wake before five. But I got through the night and cycled (yes, cycled) the 14 or so kilometres to the Medical School.

The morning was dark and warm. I had a tail wind and hardly a car went by. Despite my fears it was impossible not to feel some comfort in the sub-tropical tranquillity that cradled me.

As I walked to the hospital – a private one 20 minutes away – I began to be upset. I was plain scared of what was to come – the pain, the risk and the unconsciousness. But more than this I despaired at my powerlessness – I had opted to place myself in a situation where I knew nothing and could do nothing. I found this paradox impossibly frustrating but still I walked toward it, forcing tears away.

I arrived and sat in the foyer waiting to be admitted, observing three other equally miserable new patients with sympathy – and horror that I was one too.

I was shown to my room by an auxiliary. What I saw drove home further (as if I needed it) that despite the floral bedsheets, neat TV and new carpet, I was not booking into a hotel. They were going to cut me soon and I would be on this bed later, bleeding and hurting.

On the wall by the bed was a bag containing plastic tubes for breathing, a panel of switches with an 'emergency aid' button, and a bag holding a LIFE AID^{TM} resuscitator. Standard issue daily apparatus, trivial to a doctor or a nurse, but its presence paralysed me. How can I be here? They don't have resuscitators in hotels. There is nothing I can do now. It was agonising to lose independence so quickly and casually.

A nurse, Charleen, checked me in perfunctorily. I must have sounded scared but she was either unwilling or unable to offer me the reassurances I needed, despite my asking her as many open questions as I could think of: 'Is he a good surgeon?', 'What sort of anaesthetic will it be?' (I wanted her to say, 'Oh, a 100% safe one, you'll love it'), 'How many ops does he do at this hospital?' As we were completing the consent forms the surgeon entered. I stood up and made as if to shake hands, a gesture he either did not recognise or chose to ignore. 'Have you still got the lump?' he asked, presumably in jest. 'You know I have', I replied half in annoyance and half-bemused. He then took out his purple marker, drew a ring around the lump and started to leave.

'Is that it?' I spluttered incredulously.

He stopped. He was slowed anyway by the tight squeeze between Charleen and the wall of my room. Charleen also looked at him, unintentionally forcing him to take a step back toward me. I moved back too, so I could face him squarely.

I can't remember if he said anything. I think he probably didn't. But I know I managed to say – straight out and again with a courage that surprised me, 'What about the biopsy? What was the result of the biopsy?' I can't recall the exact words but he indicated, brusquely, that it was OK.

'So it was a pleomorphic adenoma?' I offered.

'Yes.'

'So I don't have cancer?'

'No.'

'Well that's something good at least.'

And at that he left, with a flabby wave and a 'catch you later'.

◆

It may be that this was an exceptional experience. But there was every reason for the surgeon to behave all the better with me since he knew I lecture in ethics. Furthermore, according to the nurses he is by no means 'the worst'. So I assume it is not exceptional. Indeed there is evidence all around that it is not – Paradigm Y has yet to take shape – and this is not good enough.

What, I would like to know, did the surgeon think he was doing? What was he trying to achieve? I hazard that he did not know what he was doing because: (a) he had no goal other than to do his surgery well (which he did and for which I am thankful); (b) he had no moral plan; (c) he had no moral reasoning skills; and (d) (worst of all) he was unaware that he has a daily theoretical, intellectual and practical challenge equally as demanding as his surgical function – though of a different kind.

I do not deny that what matters in the long term is that he did good surgery, but this is not to say that his short-term failure is therefore unimportant. For all we knew it could have been as long term as it was going to get. I could have died and my final 5 days would – in some part due to his moral negligence – have been amongst the most wretched of my life. And even though it turned out that these days were a small episode in my history, they did matter. They were important to me and my family, and they could have been happier had my doctor properly grasped what it is to work for someone's health.

And what is most shocking about this depressing state of affairs is that it is so *obviously* unacceptable. I have made this point before, I make it elsewhere in the Second Edition (and now the Third too), and no doubt I will continue to make it for years to come: the medical profession does not properly understand its role. Most doctors (and many other health professionals too) think clinical work is an end in itself – that medical activity defines its own purposes – but they are wrong.

My anaesthetist did a good job, as far as I know, and I felt no serious pain during or after the operation (though the surgeon was right about the lasting effects). This is as it should be and no doubt my surgeon was happy about this – anything less would have been unacceptable. Clearly one of the main aims of the operation was to avoid pain, to make sure that I was not disabled by this obstacle to my potential.

If the anaesthetist had failed to control my pain when it was within his power to do so then he would not have achieved a central goal of his work. Equally, and I insist on *equally* at this point, if any health worker in any respect within his capabilities fails to control a person's pain in general when it is in his power to do so, he will have failed to achieve a fundamental goal. People suffer mental pain too.

It matters profoundly that health workers act comprehensively. This is why I wrote this book in the first place, and why it is worth presenting it afresh, in the hope it will give new impetus to Paradigm Y.

The new edition

It is 10 years since I wrote *Ethics: The Heart of Health Care*, and much has changed in the meantime. If I could start from scratch today's book would scarcely resemble the original. Rewriting it has reminded me just how raw the First Edition was. When I wrote it I was young – not yet 30 when I began – excited and in a hurry. I had invented the Ethical Grid and I wanted the world to see it. I did not want to publish it in an academic journal my intended audience would never read – I wanted it in an accessible book with case studies, exercises and explanations about ethics.

I was so keen to get it out that I rushed the writing. I usually write countless drafts until I get the meaning and rhythm just so, but this book took only two. I knew I was going too fast, but it hardly seemed to matter. I thought I was a better writer than I was, but mostly it was a heady experience and I was carried away by it.

I have tried to compromise in this edition. The writing is less ambiguous, I have refined some points in the light of later work, and I have cut down the repetition (though repetition remains). In the First Edition I was aiming to guide readers step-by-step through the book, so I included summaries and reminders at regular intervals and more than once made the same point in different places. This is not always a bad thing, and I have retained some reinforcements. I have also added two further decision-making aids, adopted from *Liberating Medicine*,[27] a text-book written 3 years after *Ethics*.

The First Edition was an honest, innocent exploration, and I have done my best to retain this freshness. When I began the project I did not have answers to the questions: what is ethics? what is the relationship between health and morality? and how can philosophy help health workers with practical decision-making? I found out as I wrote. I hoped to convey this sense of quest to the reader, so I presented the book as a search – a hunt for the moral, to paraphrase the original title of Part II (in the First and Second Editions). I wanted the reader to share in the exploration – to wonder where it would lead and to attempt her own answers as she went along. It is only by engaging with philosophical problems that philosophy is learnt, so I wanted my questions to bother the reader too. I wanted them to become her problem – so she might work out her own ways forward, and could fully appreciate the Ethical Grid at the finish. I still do.

David Seedhouse
Auckland, New Zealand
September 1997

Growing Pains

Introduction

Will we ever attain ethically sensitive health care?
  As things stand:

1 Health care lacks a coherent philosophy of purpose.
2 Beneath the surface, different rationales compete for ascendancy.
3 Many practitioners recognise that health care is more than medical therapy.
4 However, the great bulk of health care remains medically focused.
5 Overburdened with technical tasks, most health professionals rarely catch more than a fleeting glimpse of the richer possibilities.

If we are ever going to do better than this we must openly acknowledge that health care is fundamentally a moral task.

In the midst of crisis

The health world is so conceptually disoriented it seems it may never achieve its moral potential. Mostly we just bumble along – continually troubled by territorial squabbles and inadequate resources – blind to the intellectual challenge that must be met if health work is to become all it can be.

Despite its practical successes, health care lacks a coherent account of its purpose.[24]

All notions of health (and so of what health care is meant to accomplish) stem from social values. Not everyone favours the same set of values, consequently different accounts of health care purpose co-exist. But which of them is the true version? Which form of health work is most ethically justifiable? Which interpretation of health ought to guide health policy and practice? How can we reach a philosophically secure decision about the aims of health care? These are fundamental questions – the crisis will carry on until they have been comprehensively addressed.

This conceptual crisis has not appeared overnight. Nor will it be resolved quickly (if ever), though there have been important developments during the past four decades. The British National Health Service (**NHS**), for instance, has become more open to non-medical innovation[28] and medical schools are increasingly keen to offer students a wider and more intellectually demanding education.[29]

These and other forces are subtly challenging the traditional view that medicine has an exclusive right to define the nature of health care.

Landmarks (1988)

Landmarks stand out in this potential health care revolution. Among the most prominent are:

- The rise in the popularity of alternative methods of treating disease and illness, several of which clash with traditional medical theories of disease.[30]
- Growing interest in holism and holistic medicine.[31]
- Acknowledgement by some clinicians that medicine must reassess the nature and causes of disease, and realistically contemplate the extent to which medical interventions are effective.[32,33]
- Recognition, in medical education and beyond, of the importance of ensuring meaning-ful communication between doctors and patients. Many medical schools now empha-sise how important it is that doctors genuinely understand patients' worries. Modern schools teach that doctors should be warm, approachable and empathic, should be able to engage in clear dialogue and – where appropriate – be capable of encouraging and helping patients to cope with their problems themselves. Of course, correct diag-nosis and appropriate prescribing are as important as ever, but this shift is fundamental nonetheless – it is an expansion of the traditional medical understanding of the point of health care, and it has wide ramifications.[34]
- Increasing awareness within the medical profession that the role of clinicians in health promotion is – at least potentially – less significant than that of politicians and environmentalists.[35]
- Impetus to include training and examinations in ethics for medical undergraduates.[36–38]
- Pressure from nurses to drag nursing courses away from the old idea of training in technique towards the additional goal of providing students with higher education in an academic setting. Of course nurse education must produce skilled and competent nurses; however, the 'new nurse' is a thoughtful carer armed with sufficient knowledge and experience to form her own judgements at work.[39]

Landmarks (1998)

The above landmarks remain, but change is slow. The health world's inability to embrace a philosophy of health means that some events which looked like landmarks in 1988 were of little significance.

In 1988 the medical establishment appeared (to me at least) more flexible than it actually was. Nurses have not been widely accepted as independent practitioners; there has – with the advent of the health manager – been some change in health service hierarchies, but if anything this has tended to narrow the focus of conventional health care;[40] health promotion has lost its way, baffled by a blizzard of rhetoric and naive idealism;[24] and moves to offer health care in the community – too often inspired by the desire to save money – have met with mixed results.[41] Academics – especially those in secure, tenured employment – might have been expected to lead the way: to dissect, explain and propose theoretically sound improvements to the often blatant irrationalities of the present systems. But too many find it more profitable to go along with the status quo, and just stop thinking when their conclusions begin to sound too dangerous.

Landmarks (2008)

The 1998 edition offered no new landmarks – I was struggling with the slowly dawning truth that change might not come as swiftly as I expected in 1988, as an idealistic, passionate and impatient young man.

My disillusionment over conventional health systems' blindness to simple philosophical truths became catharsis when my best friend died from cancer in 1998 – as can be seen from my final editorial for *Health Care Analysis* (reproduced with permission from Springer Netherlands):[42]

Death's moral sting

Yesterday my first friend died. He was 7 and I was 5 when we met, 42 when he was obliterated by an aimless cancer. His devastated wife is left to raise their two young girls alone, while the rest of us struggle to find any sense anywhere any more.

Death forces contemplation in a way nothing else can. Why am I still alive? Is there any meaning in this brutal world? How should we live in the face of nature's arbitrary slaughter? Does anything matter? We ponder these crushing questions as best we can, until life's mundane masquerade anaesthetises us again.

In the medical world death is commonplace. Staff become used to it. It is part of the job, to be dealt with along with everything else. It is never easy, but where death is routine it is impossible to experience every fatality as deeply as I feel the loss of my friend. Health workers have to stay in sight of the humdrum or become overwhelmed.

But death and suffering can become so familiar that they lose their moral sting. There is a dilemma here: to survive emotionally it is necessary to distance oneself from a constant stream of tragedy and torment. But once it becomes normal to stand apart from other people's anguish one's sensitivity is at risk.

After 14 years working with health professionals – the last six of these as editor of *Health Care Analysis (HCA)* – I fear that many in conventional health care overprotect themselves from the vale of tears, often at great cost to patients, to whom suffering is never commonplace.

I have countless examples. I describe a few below – some from my teaching practice, others from my editorial life.

(Continued)

Death's moral sting (Continued)

Student investigations

Each year, when examining fifth year students' powers of ethical thinking, I ask for reports of 'ethically interesting situations' encountered in clinical departments. As a result I have a box full of evidence that clinical competence and human sensitivity can be worlds apart.

Student 1: Secrets in oncology

'In the oncology clinic my role was observational. I met Mrs K, 32 years old, who had metastatic breast disease and was receiving palliative care. During the interview it became apparent to me that the patient didn't realize that the treatment option was not a cure and that she would die of her disease in the near future. After she left I raised this issue with the consultant, who replied "I don't tell them if they don't ask me".'

Student 2: Informed consent in ENT

'A diagnosis of malignancy had been made by means of a needle biopsy from a metastatic node in an elderly man's neck. The clinical director asked the patient what he knew of his condition. The patient told him he was anxious to know because nothing had been said. The director told him he had "a serious growth in his neck" and nothing more regarding prognosis or treatment. It struck me that everyone knew exactly what this man had except the patient himself. He had even received intensive investigation – the needle biopsy – without being told what was being looked for.

I find this situation interesting from the point of view that the law says that for any procedure there must be informed consent – which obviously wasn't obtained prior to the needle biopsy.'

Student 3: MS = poor quality of life?

'My case involves a 38-year-old woman who had multiple sclerosis (MS). She was living independently at home, with some help from her husband. She walked either on crutches or a "walker". She came to hospital with peritonitis – nothing to do with her MS.

She consented to an operation to wash out her abdomen and reconnect her bowel. She was very sick (septic) afterwards, unable to converse – the doctors wanted to move her to the intensive care ward. The intensive care consultant refused to take her on the ground of her MS – she said they do not accept people for intensive care who will not have a good quality of life afterwards (referring to the MS).

The patient stayed on our ward and died 2 days later.'

Student 4: He's a no-hoper anyway

'A 28-year-old Maori man presented at A&E with a chest injury following a car crash in which he was driving drunk. He had a small pneumothorax which didn't warrant treatment and was discharged to the police. The next day he was gaoled. In frustration he pushed his hand through a pane of glass, requiring readmission. A routine chest X-ray showed a complete deflation of his left lung which required urgent reinflation. The registrar inserted a chest drain, but thought it would make a good teaching case and got his colleagues (a registrar and a house officer) to insert, remove and reinsert the chest drain twice more.

This was a huge ethical issue for me. The registrar justified his actions by saying, "Well, he was a no-hoper anyway." But I knew it was wrong. However, it was only through deliberation that I understood why.'

Death's moral sting (Continued)

Student 5: Public bad news

'I was in an ENT clinic with eight of my fellow medical students one Friday morning. We were expected to go around to various rooms in the outpatient clinic, examine each patient and talk to them (I should mention that there was a consultant in the corridor yelling at anyone who wasn't in a consulting room with a patient).

A backup occurred. Either students had to be in a room in numbers in excess of four or out in the hallway being told off by the consultant. Many students responded to this by walking into any room where they saw other students, presumably assuming some sort of global consent from the patient.

Eventually a young man, his mother and grandmother were in a room being told about his cancer and his treatment options with no fewer than 15 other people crowded in. At one stage the grandmother offered a student her chair. It was accepted, even though this meant that the grandmother had to leave the room.'

These passages are true and unexceptional. Every year 20–30% of students divulge similar experiences.

It is surely obvious that in each case if the doctor had been the patient he would not have wanted to be treated in this manner. He would want information, he would want his doctor to be aware that 'quality of life' is a subjective judgement, he would want to be protected from pressure and ridicule. He would want kindness, compassion and empathy, and if he did not receive these he would want to know why.

So why are some doctors so unable to respond to visceral human needs? What is so hard about imagining oneself on the receiving end? We are all going to die, we all feel pain, almost all of us will become ill – and we will all need care then. What is so hard about giving it when one can?

Two worlds

Since *HCA* began in 1992 I have been painfully aware that the journal makes no difference to what happens in health care's name . . . papers that are written in the hope they might change something are studied by few if any practitioners:

> [This] frustrating experience is a product of two worlds which do not meet. One world is the still cloistered domain of academia, where intelligent ethical analysis is possible but practically useless. The other is the evermore utilitarian world of practice, ruled by politics and money and nowadays often openly scornful of careful reasoning[43]

Of course this is not an absolute divide. Not all health professionals are as insensitive as the doctors in my students' reports, and considerate plans are sometimes put into practice. However, it is undoubtedly not the case that increasing academic interest in health care ethics has made the difference its protagonists assume.[44] If anything contemporary health systems have become more inhuman than they used to be.[45]

They have certainly become more managed and as a result more prone to the pseudo-scientific fancies taught in management schools.[46] We are, for example, inundated with glossy material proclaiming that someone or other is 'working towards' mental health, when almost everything in psychiatric work is directed at the control of mental illness.[47] Drug companies chase profits unashamedly. Governments obsessed by rising costs (i.e. soaring prices caused by the selfish pursuit of commercial profit) hand over health care planning to accountants, a profession not primarily renowned for its kindness.[48] Precedent is allowed to hold sway over

(Continued)

Death's moral sting (Continued)

evidence[49] as powerful interests strive to remain in control. Health care is increasingly regarded as a business, as it always has been in countries outside northern Europe. ('The customer does not need to know any more than you want him to,' is as much ethics as the health care tradesman needs to know.[50]) Academics and practitioners alike fall into camps[51] in which *nothing* other camps say can possibly change their minds.

None of what I'm saying is the remotest bit scientific, I admit, and there are counterexamples. However, I doubt there are enough to dent the general case that our basic human experiences are being devalued. A system supposed to cater for them has become so insightless that patients are disappearing in a smog of technical efficiency. The desire to manage health systems as if they are essentially the same as business corporations – and to do so in a way that fosters anxiety and secrecy in employees – means everyday callousness is obscured so long as the required outputs are produced at the right cost. In turn, the lack of humanity of many of those at the top of coal-face hierarchies feeds a system where caring for suffering people is not seen, is not rewarded and is even discouraged if it is considered too expensive.

The answers

It is not difficult to say what ought to be done to change this frequently obscene situation, yet much of what is needed is apparently politically impossible. In order to achieve a humane health system governments should:

- Remove personal financial incentive for service provision
- Fund a comprehensive public system through progressive general taxation
- Employ salaried staff, professionally remunerated and contractually forbidden to practice privately
- Prohibit all inducements to health professionals from commercial companies, including all advertising
- Pass laws to ensure that all policy decisions are made openly by publicly accountable decision-makers
- Distinguish human helping from business dealing by developing or adopting a clear and practically explicit philosophy of practice[24]
- Encourage continuing public discussion of this philosophy
- Educate health care students broadly, in the humanities as well as the sciences
- Insist on in-service training in comprehensive ethical analysis[52]

Remember death's moral sting

But above all the answer is never to forget death's moral sting. There are two ways to go. The dominant path just now is to become progressively numb in the face of stupid policy, arrogant practice and relentless human annihilation. The alternative – immeasurably more noble, and our saving grace – is to feel death's moral sting all the time. It is all around us. The solution to health care's failings is to use human suffering to provoke humane thinking. Death can make us dull, or it can reawaken us to the importance of every single human interaction every single minute. If death has a lesson it is that life is short, precious and every last bit of it matters to someone we can touch now.

To the memory of Andrew John Richardson ('Rickers') 1955–1998

The 2008 edition has no new landmarks either – however, the controlled anger of my editorial has grown into a quieter, practical realism: yes, the medical establishment holds as much power as ever; yes, philosophically empty habits will continue to shape health care's future BUT change will come too, and with the advent of new communication technologies is now a lot more likely than it used to be (as you can see from **Chapter Eleven**).

The health world is changing

The idea that it is desirable to provide health care solely according to clinical priorities (ignoring social and moral aspirations) is under pressure. Medicine has dominated orthodox health care because of its high social status and hefty financial muscle, and because its practitioners have privileged knowledge. But although health work appears as controlled by medicine as ever, beneath the surface inspirational conceptual and practical developments are taking shape, even though the majority of health workers are still not aware of them.

Thomas Kuhn's theory of paradigms

Thomas Kuhn's theory of paradigm change is a handy way to illustrate this (though I do not claim that paradigms are real).[53]

Kuhn was interested in the history of scientific research. He investigated the attitudes and beliefs of research scientists and found that for most of the time – usually for their entire careers – most scientists have common aims, accept the same standards and procedures, and embrace shared criteria of success. They engage in what he calls 'normal science', where they try to solve 'puzzles' – or technical difficulties – within an accepted tradition. Occasionally scientists are faced with a crisis that causes them to question the most basic assumptions of their research tradition. When this happens what was thought to be bedrock can turn to quicksand, and everything is thrown into uncertainty.

During a paradigm change events and results of experiments are observed for which the current set of explanations (the present paradigm) is unable to account, a phenomenon accompanied by a growing perception that the existing way of seeing things is inadequate. This perception – that 'there is something profoundly wrong about the theoretical framework in which we are working' – can develop into an intellectual crisis resolvable only by redefining the entire project. Such redefinition is impossible until the most politically powerful researchers have become convinced it must be done.

A classic example of paradigm shift

The change in perspective when Newton's theory of mechanics was superseded by modern physics is often cited as a classic example of a paradigm shift or scientific revolution. Newton's theoretical structure was applied fruitfully for over two centuries.[54] However, as developments in technology both demanded and facilitated increasingly precise measurements and predictions, Newtonian mechanics was found not quite accurate enough. It was discovered to be impossible to increase accuracy further within the tradition. Instead Newton's mechanics was supplanted by another theory, which explained the evidence in a radically different way. This was not a steady progression but a dramatic upheaval – a remarkable revolution in thinking. The implication of this for our understanding of the nature of science is immense since it calls into question the 'common-sense' that science is a steadily accumulating body of public knowledge about reality.

After studying similar historical examples it seemed to Kuhn that 'common-sense' is mistaken, and that spectacular changes in direction can and do take place within well-established research disciplines, even those that have achieved considerable practical success. Newton's stature as a scientist and original thinker is unshakeable, yet modern physicists no longer build on his physical theories. Good research can be done that produces fundamentally mistaken hypotheses, so progress in science cannot only be a matter of adding to existing work. Sometimes accepted theories and wisdoms have to be rejected. And this process can happen in all research traditions, not just in natural science.

Many philosophers disagree with Kuhn, arguing that it is both arbitrary and melodramatic to call a series of explicable developments a 'revolution'. Some critics point out that if the history of science is studied with care there are always strands of continuity to be found.[55]

While Kuhn's theory of paradigm change clearly does not provide a complete explanation of the growth of scientific thought, it is nevertheless illustrative to explore his idea in relation to contemporary health care. To do so is inevitably to over-simplify, but it can help show how the idea of paradigm change might encourage a more complete appreciation of health care change.

The heart of the crisis in health care

A 'paradigm shift' looks like this:

Figure 20 The paradigm shift in the abstract

Paradigm X represents the old consensus, and Y its successor. The overlap symbolises the common ground remaining. So far as the classic example is concerned, Newton and his contemporaries can be thought of as working in Paradigm X. When it was discovered that Newtonian mechanics could not explain some astronomical observations this paradigm was thrown into crisis and a new one eventually assumed dominance. In physics Paradigm Y, which inspired relativity theory, the uncertainty principle and quantum mechanics,[56] was a radical departure from Paradigm X. Many of its basic assumptions contradicted Newtonian theory, although some beliefs were still shared. For instance, the use of logic and mathematics, the demand that all theories should be tested as rigorously as possible, and the terminology of the old paradigm, remained common.[55] In other words, even when a radical shift occurs the two spheres are not totally separate. Some philosophers of science maintain that the shift is neither as neat nor as simple as the Venn diagram illustration suggests, and that it usually makes more sense to think of the new paradigm as encompassing the old one, retaining the 'falsified knowledge' and mistaken beliefs, but finding this information of little or no relevance to future work:

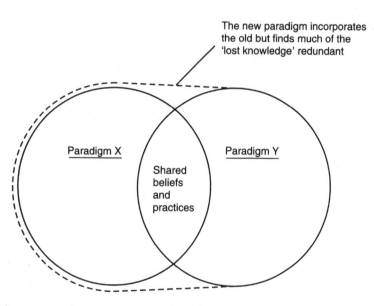

Figure 21 The new paradigm encompassing the old one

Relevance to health care

The idea of paradigm change is a helpful analogy in the world of health care. Of course, even this very general idea is not wholly appropriate, since health care is more to do with practice than research, and Kuhn's interest lay mostly with scientific theorising. Nevertheless there is a partial correspondence.

The present situation in health care might be caricatured like this.

Paradigm X

Paradigm X contains the 'old school' of health care where health is thought to be nothing more than the state of a person not suffering from disease, illness or infirmity; where the medical profession defines its rationale without consulting those whom it seeks to serve; where the idea of medical education is that as many facts as possible should be crammed by students (who soon come to see their 'education' instrumentally – something to be got through to become a doctor); where the idea of providing students with a proper grounding in ethics is seen as pointless – or worse, seen as a threat; where technical decisions are made 'for the good of the patients' without patients' involvement; where patients are used to test the effect of drug treatments in controlled experiments without their knowledge; where patients are not permitted to see their medical records; where the health service is organised in strict hierarchical lines in which everyone knows his or her place; where curing disease through clinical science is the primary motivation; and where measures of success or failure in the care of patients are predominantly quantifiable, emphasising severity of disease, degree of deviation from statistical norms and life expectancy.

Paradigm Y

Paradigm Y is the fruition of the developments and initiatives listed (see pp. 4–5 in the First Edition, pp. 23–24 in the Second Edition, p. 2 in this edition), plus other practical improvements. It is based on a different theoretical understanding of work for health – its impetus is the simple idea that people are of fundamental consequence. In Paradigm Y curing disease and illness and increasing the length of life remain important, but are not always as important as increasing the autonomy of those who request or need health care, distributing available resources fairly, education and (at least sometimes) respecting people's choices even if they conflict with given advice.

Paradigm Y policy-makers understand that health in the richest sense can be more to do with personal freedom than physical fitness. Its health services are organised to ensure all workers have a say in what happens to it; the users of the service are allowed to see whatever has been written about them and, as far as circumstances permit, are involved in all decisions that affect them. The task of enabling people to develop mentally, physically and emotionally – creatively throughout their lives – is a primary motivation (see Figure 22), necessitating a restructuring of most services.

Paradigm Y harnesses web-based technology, not just to improve clinical management systems but to include professionals and patients emotionally and socially. Paradigm Y information systems share values, feelings and human reasoning at least as well and at least as extensively as they share electronic medical records (see **Chapter Eleven**).

Paradigm Y has not yet crystallised – though its outline is visible to those who know how to look.

A hidden crisis?

Many in the health world do not accept Kuhn's image has anything to do with health care. Any evidence of a conceptual and practical health care 'crisis' is at best superficial,

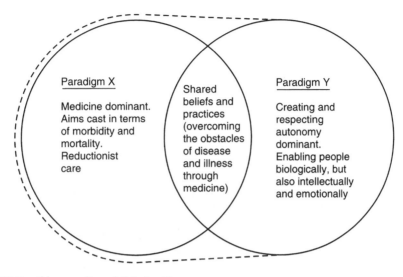

Figure 22 Possible paradigm shift in health care

they will say. The conventional position is that there have been some changes of emphasis, and some secondary developments which complement the main body of medical work. But slow evolution hardly constitutes intellectual crisis, and clinical medicine rightly governs health work.

These critics might be right – Paradigm Y may turn out to be nothing more than wishful thinking. However, it is worth remembering that during his investigation into the history of scientific research Kuhn noticed that during the 'crisis period' – the time when two paradigms are competing for ascendancy – only very few people recognise that a transition is taking place. Some may suspect a revolution, but it is only with hindsight that the true extent of the crisis becomes apparent.

It would not be too surprising if the current foment were to escape the attention of busy health workers absorbed in particular tasks. There is little enough time for them to reflect on changes even within their own disciplines. Standing back to take a view of health care as a whole can appear impossible to those daily involved in dealing with the many distressing obstacles that hinder patients. And it is necessary to learn of a great many disparate developments to have anything like an informed understanding of what is going on. As with political revolutions, for all of us working during the transition, it may only be when the dust has settled that we will see the complete picture.

The gestalt-switch

Kuhn uses a further image to back his claim. He argues that the change of perception that happens when an individual notices he is working in a new paradigm can be likened to a 'gestalt-switch', an idea derived from the Gestalt school of psychology which flourished at the start of the twentieth century.[57]

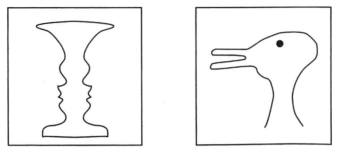

Vase or profiles?　　　　　　　　A duck or a rabbit?

Figure 23 Examples of the gestalt-switch

The gestalt-switch is famously illustrated by showing that an arrangement of lines on paper can be seen in different ways. The pictures in Figure 23 might be either a duck or a rabbit, and either a vase or two faces, according to what we think we are seeing.

There are two points worth noting here: first that the theories we have about what we are observing help us make sense of what we observe, and second that it is necessary to have a relevant theory in order to make sense of anything. Kuhn's insight was to extrapolate this idea into the realm of science where if we hold one theory (say Newtonian mechanics) we 'see' the evidence in one way, yet if we hold an alternative theory (say the new theory of physics) we 'see' precisely the same evidence in a different way.

It is – I hope – not over-stretching the point to develop this line of thought in a way germane to the future of health care. The theories we hold about our everyday work – the subjective theoretical framework in which we each operate – obviously affects our interpretation of the world, and what we do in it. Health workers' understanding of their practice affects both their performance and their attitude towards those for whom they are caring. So – since a great variety of subjective understandings exist – it is surely important to make them overt – to reveal them to their holders as they really are (which is what the Values Exchange and Health Exchange try to do – see **Chapter Eleven**). Once this is routinely done, health workers will see that beliefs they take to be self-evident are not obvious at all (they will see a range of plausible alternatives) and it may then also be possible to shape future developments to correspond with the foundations theory of health, by highlighting the most creative interpretations of health work.

Health workers can create future change through present practice

What health workers do now – in everyday practice – is instrumental in bringing about the future of health care.

We are constantly faced with choices which may shape our destiny. Our paths are limited by what we have done, by our talents, our education, our circumstances and the historical era in which we live, but we almost always have some choice about what to do, what to believe, how to act towards others and what to say. Even in circumstances where our choices are restricted, alternatives are usually open to us. For instance, a teacher may have no choice but to teach a class of disinterested and unruly teenagers, but still have significant options about how best to deal with them. And even where choice appears totally limited we can at least choose between doing and not doing a thing. We can create ourselves, more than we think. And just as we can create ourselves, through our actions we can create conditions in which other people are better placed to create more fulfilled versions of themselves too.

To bring about the paradigm transition, it is absolutely crucial that health workers not only speak of 'positive health' and 'empowering' but act according to richer ideas of health. If the new paradigm is to triumph, health workers who want it to be reality must ensure they are true to themselves, and that their actions match their beliefs.

Disease or health? The greatest frustration

The gestalt-switch analogy also helps explain the central, frustrating tension which is currently preventing the paradigm shift. Gestalt-switch difficulties can be overcome, and the way to do it is to display and explain both options simultaneously. This should not be so difficult. Do you want to see just the one thing – either a duck or a rabbit – or do you want to be able to say, 'I see them both. Now I can make up my mind which I prefer'?

Clarification of meaning is crucial

Clarification of meaning can make a real difference to what is done. If work for health is only taken to mean work to cure disease then the implications for practice are massively different from those that follow if work for health is taken to mean 'liberating all human potential to the fullest degree'. In an earlier book,[8] various meanings and theories of health were discussed, among them the views that 'health is a state of complete physical, social and mental well-being, not merely the absence of disease, illness and infirmity'; the theory that health occurs when disease is absent; the theory that a person is healthy if she can perform her normal social function; and the theory that health is a strength – an ability to cope with or adapt to the problems life throws in people's paths. These theories are not fully compatible with each other. They will not gel into a coherent whole without contradiction. For example, a person might have a disease (and so be unhealthy according to one possible meaning of health) and yet still be able to perform her normal social function (and so be healthy according to an alternative meaning of health).

The analysis offered in *Health: The Foundations for Achievement* revealed a common theme beneath the various theories. This is that work for health is always designed to remove obstacles in the path of biological, intellectual, emotional and creative human potentials. The *Foundations* argument is that health is a richer idea than commonly supposed – health is to do with human flourishing, not merely the absence of disease. Effort against disease can be genuine health work, but it is not the whole story.

Once you understand the *Foundations* analysis it is very hard to see why this is not completely obvious to everyone. For example, consider the hypothetical job title 'Health Promotion and Disease Prevention Officer'. No-one would dispute that this title makes sense, so everyone should be able to see that the use of two separate terms – 'health promotion' and 'disease prevention' – implies different meanings.

Much of the ambiguity in health studies has come about (and remains) because this major distinction seems invisible to most people. Forward-looking authors writing about health frequently introduce nebulous ideas like 'positive health' and 'well-being' to indicate that health is not one side of a see-saw counterbalanced by disease and illness. But then, having glimpsed one picture momentarily – having realised that the duck can also be a rabbit – even the most radical health promotion visionaries slip back into the old habit of discussing how to decrease disease and illness.

Health writers and workers caught in the trap fleetingly realise that health is to do with fulfilment, but then they hit a daunting mental block. As soon as they begin to consider how this fulfilment can be made concrete, they fall under the spell of medicine again, hurtled backwards as if attached to a piece of elastic stretched as far as it can go.

The basic problem is that health is still habitually thought of from a point of reference that begins with disease. This is such a powerful idea that almost everyone seems to think that when talking about health you must necessarily refer to disease, illness, handicap and injury sooner or later – or else you cannot be talking about health at all.

Health promoters continually insist that health is more than the absence of disease and illness, yet their official work is almost entirely directed at preventing disease and illness. Having experienced a fleeting insight into the fullest sense of health the very next thought of the ensnared health educator is always something like, 'How can I persuade this person to adopt the kind of habits which will make him less prone to becoming ill?' Certainly, if a health educator can achieve this particular goal then she stands a good chance of enhancing a person's life in general (for instance, if the person who is the target of the persuasion avoids a stroke as a result then this will prevent a wide range of obstacles, not just brain damage *per se*). But the trouble is that constant emphasis on ameliorating disease and illness in the name of health embalms a central mistake – the continuation of the unreflective assumption that preventive and curative medicine is the best means of helping an adult person to become more of what she could be. Yet of course it is not. Health is not only a matter for medicine and can be created and improved in numerous ways for which medicine has no brief.

Summary

Chapter One is not much different from the way it was 20 years ago. It still argues:

1 The health care world does not have to be the way it is – despite the engrained tradition, status and money involved. There are better ways to think about and practice health care
2 The purpose of health care is not immutable. The idea that health is nothing more than the opposite of disease is just one amongst several meaningful inspirations for health care practice
3 Within establishment health care there is much activity that draws on richer theories of health. Some of it even contradicts strictly medical goals

Summary (Continued)

4 If enough of this 'deviant' activity can rise to the surface there will be a paradigm shift, or at the very least more and more people will begin to think of health care differently, and will come to expect additional support from their health carers

5 It is up to those health workers who prefer a richer, autonomy-based ethos, to express the new paradigm in what they do. Pretty much everything hinges on how health workers think and act right now.

The next chapter is an attempt to accelerate change by showing that ethics is the key – it simply makes logical and ethical sense to see human autonomy as the heart of health care rather than to think curing disease, injury and handicap is all there is.

Health work is moral work. Consequently, by making clear the range and importance of the moral content of health work, by bringing what already exists to the fore in its proper focus, it should be possible to bring about the most desirable form of the new paradigm. Ethics is the key to the formation of health work's new era.

Ethics is the Key

Introduction

How can health professionals come to see the richer possibilities of health care? How can we create an ethically sensitive health care industry?

The answer is to understand ethics properly, and that means recognising that ethics is everywhere, and personal.

There are many different approaches to ethics. This chapter distinguishes between everyday and technical ethics, and briefly introduces some elements of technical ethics.

The ultimate aim of both approaches should be to encourage thought about the social and philosophical sources of ethical dilemmas.

Once health professionals understand the extent of the ethical iceberg – once they realise that ethics is everywhere – they possess the ethical key to the new paradigm.

Most people regard ethics as a secondary concern in health and medical work. Some even believe that ethical issues are not relevant at all.[58] But they're wrong: ethics is the key to release thoughtful health workers from the present over-technical paradigm.

Work for health is a moral endeavour

The slogan 'work for health is a moral endeavour' is a helpful reminder of the fundamental connection between intervening to improve other people's health and engaging in ethical activity. Logically, whenever anyone tries to help someone with a health problem they must attempt to remove an obstacle of some kind (it doesn't matter whether the obstacle is clinical, emotional, social or something else). As they attempt to remove the obstacle they are firmly in the moral realm because their intervention is meant to affect the life of at least one other person. This is the essence of ethical engagement – the health worker has to think about what she wants to achieve and how she wants to achieve it, and she must consider whether the person she is trying to help has the same goals (she is likely to achieve this by comparing her rational fields with her client's – see

Introduction). To work for health in a meaningful way the health worker must engage in a personal, contextual, ethical reflection.

While it is impossible to say definitively that work for health is a particular, specific type of moral endeavour, it is vital to remember that health work is always a moral endeavour of some kind – health care is never ever a matter of evidence alone.

What is ethics?

(Note: in this book no distinction is made between 'ethics' and 'morality'. All variations of each word are used interchangeably.)

If you want to understand the importance of ethics, you should first be clear what ethics is not – ethics is not a single body of knowledge about what is right and wrong and it is not something that anyone can be expert in. Yes, people can study for degrees in technical ethical theory but this does not make them any more or less ethical in everyday life. Our social world is far more intricate and enigmatic than this.

Because ethical reflection is meant to give answers to questions about how men and women should act, the scope of ethical concern is infinitely varied. This diversity can be dissected into many different types, the analysis of which can become very complicated (as any survey of texts in moral philosophy will show) since most types contain a host of further sub-divisions (see **Chapter Six**). These distinctions can be interesting to professional philosophers and their students, who enjoy debating their respective merits, but they have little impact on daily life.

To see this, compare *everyday* and *technical* ethics.

Everyday ethics

We all, at one time or another, discuss moral issues. Such encounters happen daily: at work, in supermarket queues, in bars and cafes, on trains, at bus stops – everywhere people are interested and concerned enough to discuss issues affecting human life and relationships. Typically, participants express their approval of various values and principles and argue that these should be followed by other people (sometimes they even follow them themselves). Most people's positions are not the result of thorough philosophical analysis, and from time to time we all advocate ideas that are either inconsistent with one another, or which contradict those for which we have argued previously. This unpredictability is acceptable at the level of casual conversation – in everyday ethics – but is studiously avoided in technical ethics.

One example of everyday ethics

Different people's everyday ethics can vary immensely, both in content and consistency. Usually only limited attention is paid to overall coherence, and it is common for everyday ethical decisions to be taken according to 'the moment' – according to the context and emotional state of a particular person at a particular time. Even for the same individual, different circumstances can give rise to different, even paradoxical, ethical intuitions. Consider, for example, one possible 'system' of everyday ethics, held by Carolyn Smith.

Carolyn's everyday ethical outlook is based on a simple set of dictums that can – sometimes – give coherent answers to human problems. She believes: 'it is wrong to be underhand and deceitful at work', 'people who look after number one should be respected', 'you should always respect the wishes of other people' and 'you should take only what a job is worth'.

On the face of it this looks a plausibly consistent ethical outlook. But – in social context – there are problems even with this simple *raison d'être*. Carolyn is a neonatal nurse who respects an ambitious consultant (because he is very good at looking after number one). She discovers that the doctor is using robust physiotherapy experimentally on newborns, against the wishes of some of the parents (consequently her framework is immediately found wanting: she cannot respect everyone's wishes simultaneously – though he is looking after 'number one' the doctor wants to continue the experiment while the parents want Carolyn to stop him).

It does not usually require sustained investigation of any given everyday ethics to find contradiction – if a consistent ethical position is desired then something more than *ad hoc* frameworks and comfortable intuition is needed.

Technical ethics

Technical ethics sets out to avoid the vagaries of everyday ethics, but has to pay a different price – technical ethicists have to sacrifice flexibility and realism for the sake of technical coherence.

It is the (self-appointed) job of moral philosophers to devise and refine technical ethical theory. They try to design theories that are internally consistent, and which contain principles and notions that complement each other.

Aspects of technical ethics

Technical ethics can be divided into various aspects. Different analysts have devised many different classifications. Three of these – *moral philosophy as a quest to understand 'the good'*, *moral philosophy based on consequences or duties* and *moral philosophy as a process of deliberation* – are probably the most well-known.

1 Moral philosophy as a quest to understand 'the good'

One branch of technical ethics does not tackle practical ethical problems directly. Instead it seeks to understand the nature of 'goodness' itself – its advocates argue that it is only by first understanding what goodness means that anyone can aim to be good.

It is possible to become so preoccupied with questions of meaning that it is only meaning – and nothing else – that is seen as the problem. So, two points need to be borne in mind. First, it is undoubtedly crucial in any serious inquiry that the meanings of key terms are clarified as far as possible. But second, it must not be thought that, merely by clarifying the meanings of words, real problems in the real world can be solved. The clarification of meaning is an essential part of inquiry into ethics, but it is only a part.

Good

For example, in order to work out what it is good to do it is important to stress that the word 'good' has at least three separate meanings.

a. *'Good' as a description of objects that are useful.* People talk of a 'good clock' or a 'good motor car' using this sense of 'good'. Used in this way 'good' is often ethically neutral, at least when it is used to describe a physical function per se (this is a good clock because it tells the time accurately, which is what it is supposed to do: this is a good car because I can rely on it to start in the morning). Of course, if one asks: 'what is this good (i.e. functionally efficient) car being used FOR?' then one is asking for an answer with moral content. For example, the car might be being used by a volunteer to transport disabled people to day centres, or it might be a getaway car for armed robbers, and there is usually felt to be a moral difference between these two purposes.

b. *'Good' as a description of things that are pleasing or enjoyable in themselves.* Using 'good' in this sense, it is possible to describe an aesthetically pleasing painting, or a productive garden, as good in an ethically neutral way – though even here there can be ethical content.

c. *'Good' used to describe the specifically moral.* When the word 'good' is used like this it describes human activity – usually human activity that affects other people, not only the actor. This use of the word has close connections with other moral words such as 'ought', 'right', 'just' and 'duty'. It is frequently asserted, for instance, that a person ought to do what is good.

Such assertions are never ethically neutral. They are always based on human preferences (values) about what we think is morally good.

2 Moral philosophy based on either consequences or duties

Most students of moral philosophy are quickly introduced to two different approaches to ethical reasoning: working out how to act according to the likely consequences of actions, and working out how to act according to moral duties.

By way of introduction to this pivotal debate – enlarged in **Chapter Six** – consider these traditional examples.

Consequences

One famous technical ethical theory is known as *utilitarianism*. Generally speaking, utilitarians assess the morality of people's actions by looking either at the actual results (and so judging morality in retrospect) or by calculating likely future consequences. For utilitarians the best (most moral) actions are those that produce the most favourable balance of good over bad. So the worth of any action – whether it is a small kindness to another person, or a decision to declare war on a nation – is considered to be moral or immoral dependent on whether or not the outcome is a balance of human happiness over misery (at least according to one version of utilitarianism).

Duties
The (supposedly) competing version of technical ethics is *deontology*. According to this outlook what matters most is not the result but the fact that a person acted according to a perceived duty. For example, an advocate of deontology might argue that certain principles, truth-telling and promise-keeping perhaps, are fundamental to morality and that, to be moral, a person has an obligation always to abide by them – whatever the consequences. Even if the outcome of telling the truth will produce more misery than happiness, to tell it – to abide by preconceived moral duty – is the right and honest way to act.

3 Moral philosophy as a process of deliberation

This third form of technical ethics makes ultimate plea neither to rules nor to past and future consequences. This variety – moral philosophy as a deliberative process – is part of the approach advocated in this book.

The essence of deliberative ethics is consideration of the best ways to create more of what might be in oneself and others: Aristotle called this goal 'eudaimonia' (meaning happiness or flourishing). This version of moral reasoning is impossible to those who believe that being ethical is a question of following specific rules and codes of conduct, or of always acting according to a specific view of what is right and wrong.

Aristotle thought deliberation was the essence of ethics, since a contemplative process must be undertaken in every case where there are decisions to be made about the worth of human activity. He divided knowledge into three different disciplines: theoretical, practical and productive.[59] The majority of his works were concerned with his 'theoretical' category: 'natural science' – where 'natural and regular laws' apply. According to Aristotle, there is no need for deliberation under this heading because this is the realm of fact, of mathematical law and of predictable physical cause and effect (see my use of the 'just is' category in the Introduction).

But ethics is different. In ethical matters there is not the certainty of natural science. Rather there is an infinite variety of human circumstances and situations, and there can be no universal laws or sets of principles that can be applied to every situation. Whatever rule is invented in moral philosophy, sooner or later there will be a case in which it will be better to break it in order to create a more desirable human potential. And because of this it is far better – far more moral – to enhance human judgement in the uncertain field of human action and interaction, rather than to instil imperfect sets of rules in people, as if these rules are inviolable commandments. Rules and principles are useful to the deliberative process, but subjective judgement in context is ultimate.

Ethics and the tip of the iceberg

Though these aspects of technical ethics are commonly discussed in ethics textbooks, they merely skim the surface of what it is to be ethical. You can study as many ethical theories and texts as you like, but unless you can see the components of ethical thinking in context and in the raw, you will never get better at it – this is the message of the Third Edition – it does no harm to inform yourself about ethical theory, nor does it hurt to study difficult social situations you might encounter in your work – but don't confuse this with systematic personal reflection and sustained interest in the views and values of others, which is ultimately what ethics is about.

A practical, constructive distinction

A good way to understand the nature and the limits of conventional ethics is to distinguish between **dramatic** or **specific ethics, persisting ethics** and **ethics in a general sense**, and then to recognise that everything in the social world sits inside the iceberg in Figure 24: ethics is everywhere.

Dramatic ethics

The term 'specific/dramatic ethics' (hereafter 'dramatic ethics') refers to matters that seem to stand self-contained, in isolation from other personal or work issues. Dramatic ethics are hard choices. For example, a doctor has a dramatic ethical problem when she wonders whether she ought to discontinue ventilating a dying patient in order to transplant organs to three waiting recipients, or whether she should continue treatment because of the slim possibility the patient might regain consciousness.

In this sort of situation a decision has to be made – one way or another. Having assessed the various pros and cons, all that's required is the courage to say – specifically – yes or

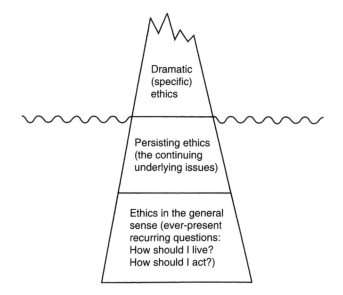

Figure 24 Ethics and the tip of the iceberg – a broad distinction between different types of ethics

no. Dramatic ethics is the domain of the 'tragic choice', where any choice comes with an unwanted price. Because dramatic ethical problems usually have lurid appeal – and tend to excite the makers of television documentaries – news-media focus on dramatic ethics has led to (or has reinforced) the now commonplace perception that such 'hot spots' are all there is to ethics. But, really, ethical dilemmas are nothing more than ethics at the tip of the iceberg.

Persisting ethics

Because it is much easier – and more entertaining – to think of ethics as 'either/or decision-making', there is never enough attention paid to 'persisting ethics' – the issues that permanently underlie the intermittent ethical dramas. For example, behind the specific question: 'should abortion be a legal right?' there are constant, philosophically fundamental, questions about what it is to be a person or potential person, the degree of control a woman ought to have over what happens to her body and the nature of a moral right.

Ethics in the general sense

The phrase 'ethics in the general sense' refers to deliberation about how best to conduct one's life in general. The person who deliberates in this general sense of ethics realises that all thought and action can and should be the subject of moral reflection. Admittedly it might not be instantly obvious that decisions about whether or not to pass the salt to a fellow diner, or whether or not to continue sitting in an armchair doing nothing, have moral relevance – but they do in this general sense (see the discussion of Ethical A and B in the **Introduction to the Second Edition** for a more complete explanation).

To see the point of 'ethics in the general sense' all you need understand is that whatever one does, either to oneself or another person, does not have to be done. Alternative courses of action are almost always possible, and these alternatives can be valued differently and can have different consequences. Dependent upon what you choose to do, you can always enhance or damage your own or someone else's existence, even if only to a small extent.

To take the examples mentioned above: if you are asked to pass the salt at a dinner party you can do this gladly, casually or with obvious irritation – possibly causing the person who made the request to feel more or less at ease. The result of a positive behaviour might be that the recipient will enjoy his meal more, be stimulated into interesting conversation and you will probably have had a beneficial effect on all the diners. Alternatively, if you know something about nutrition and heart disease you might decide to inform your friend of the possible consequences of excessive consumption of salt. You might tell him this nonchalantly, jokingly or seriously – you might even choose to scare him and cause him to feel guilty and anxious about his past habits.

And if you are sitting in an armchair – well, you might be doing something else. In normal circumstances there should, of course, be no compulsion on a person not to sit in an armchair if that is what he chooses. However, the inescapable fact is that other things are possible. By remaining in the armchair (say you just happen to have woken up in it, you don't need to relax any more and you simply continue to do nothing) you are doing little or nothing to create more of the possibilities open to yourself, nor are you doing anything to enable other people. It's hardly the depth of immorality to remain in an armchair (everyone has to be somewhere, after all) but neither is it the height of morality. You could be doing more. Whether or not to sit in an armchair is a moral issue.

Two illustrations of the iceberg distinctions

1 The 1982 conflict between Britain and Argentina over the Falkland Islands (or Malvinas) (ancient history for anyone under 35) is a good illustration of the iceberg.

The conflict flared quickly and was soon over. It focused intense interest in some quarters on dramatic ethical issues. There was, for instance, widespread discussion about the morality of killing hundreds of people over a relatively barren and sparsely populated island; about whether the principle of 'sovereignty' should take precedence over the principle of 'common humanity'; about whether any nation has a clear and certain duty to protect her citizens wherever they might be; and about whether blatant lying and secrecy, by a democratically elected government in 'communication' with the general public, was ethically correct even in time of war. (Some of these are also 'persistent' issues – the iceberg distinctions are illustrative, not clear-cut.)

Although the dramatic issues associated with the Falklands War are no longer in the limelight, they and other ethically striking dilemmas sit at the iceberg's summit during every war (for example, depressingly similar issues erupted when it was discovered that Britain and the USA had invaded Iraq on the apparently false assumption that Iraq was building 'weapons of mass destruction').[60]

Lying below sea level, at the next level down, are persisting ethical questions which existed before, during and after the Falklands conflict (and every other war). These are at least as important as the dramatic ones, even though they are not so immediately apparent. Is it moral to maintain a large army in peace time when the social and environmental conditions of millions of citizens are self-evidently debilitating? Should the public have access to more information about the workings of the military? Should pacifists have the right to refuse to pay taxation to maintain armed forces? Should governments elected by a minority of votes have the right to call upon everyone to go to war?

Ethics in the general sense is depicted at the base of the iceberg (Figure 24) but in truth it permeates the whole edifice. Yet it is hard for us to see life like this, so we rarely focus on ethics in the general sense. We become aware of this part of the iceberg only when we think of ethics as a personal task, as we do when we ask such questions as, 'What can I do about these dramatic and persisting issues?' 'Should I campaign to put over my point of view?' 'Should I distort evidence to persuade people of my position?' 'If I am with a group of relative strangers, perhaps in a pub after a few drinks, all of whom vehemently support a position to which I am strongly opposed, should I explain what I believe or should I let it pass?' Such questions are no less hard to answer than those raised in the rest of the iceberg. In fact, they are almost always the hardest of all.

2 Because ethics in the general sense is such a feature of human life (like the air we breath) we tend not to realise that we are constantly faced with ethical situations: as a rule we do not examine most of what we do. We just do what we do and get used to and it becomes routine. However, once we become aware of the extent of ethics in a general sense, we recognise the true magnitude of our responsibilities. Of course we would be made insane if we reflected ethically on everything, nor can anyone do very much about most of life's injustices – not even those which trouble us greatly. However, to know ethics in the general sense is constantly to be aware of the tension between duty and inertia – a tension between doing what one ought to, and going along with things as they are.

When I was writing the Second Edition of this book I became acutely aware of how easy it is to shirk responsibility, even though I knew I should frequently ask myself 'How should I act?', 'How should I live?', 'What should I do for the moral best?' I was a lecturer in a Medical School, and had been in the job for long enough to have a list as long as my arm of all that was not right at the School (see the Introduction) – and yet I was doing nothing very much about it, justifying my policy on utilitarian grounds (I told myself it was better that I'm around to teach the undergraduates).

I knew of many patients who were being treated shabbily yet I did nothing to help them. I continually came across dramatic ethical issues (most commonly – patients not being properly informed of their conditions, not for resuscitation notes placed almost arbitrarily, and rationing decisions made covertly, according to social and ethnic criteria) each of which raised central, persisting questions. I knew, from what I understood of ethics in the general sense, that it is not enough to shrug and say: 'What can I do? . . . it is too big for me' – for I could have done all sorts of things if I had chosen to. But I did not because I was sure the consequences were unlikely to be good for me, or for the reputation of ethics teaching in the School.

At the time of writing the Second Edition I was deeply troubled by a patient who had been kept in a secure mental illness unit for 2 years. The circumstances that led to her incarceration were certainly dramatic – she was arrested and accused of repeated intimidation; she screamed her protests in the cells; she was committed involuntarily for psychiatric treatment; she was diagnosed 'erotomanic' (amongst other things); she said she was a witch; and she had consistently failed to respond to treatment in the ways her medical guardians wanted (she would not, for instance, ever agree that she was mentally ill despite enormous pressure on her to 'confess' to this).

The persisting issues are far too numerous to list fully, though they include questions about the nature of mental illness; psychiatric taxonomy; the point of involuntary treatment (is it to cure, to restrain or to protect others?); competence (the patient was extremely clear about what had happened to her and to a lay person seemed normally competent); the relationship between criminal responsibility and insanity; the motivations of psychiatrists; and the clash between cultural outlooks (the patient's family and her ancestors were witches too).

Ethics in the general sense required me to consider how best to act in this case. I thought: should I do nothing? Should I work subtly behind the scenes by speaking with her psychiatrists – most of whom I knew a little? Should I advocate for her more openly? Or should I try to publicise her case in the press? Whatever I chose I knew this was not only an issue for her – it was an ethical issue for me too.

After doing nothing for 2 years – other than feel guilty – I decided that I had to get involved. I began to work with her solicitor on her case. I visited her. I read her notes. I closely examined how the system had been treating her.

I found her to be a strange person, with very strong beliefs about who she was and about social rights and wrongs. I could not judge whether she was mentally ill since I do not understand the concept – however, I read the psychiatric textbooks and I could see why her psychiatrists used the categories they did and why they were detaining her. But I could also see her point of view, and I could see that on her own terms at least, she was a solidly rational person.

She argued with great consistency that she was a witch, that the person she was accused of stalking had in fact been in a relationship with her, that he attacked her first, that she was not a danger to anyone and that she was definitely not mentally ill. I could also see from her notes that she had been given a wide range of diagnoses over the years and that at one stage her psychiatrists had written that they had reached the point where they had no idea what diagnosis was appropriate. It was also recorded that she had received every powerful antipsychotic in the doctors' armoury, yet this had not changed her mental state one iota (though she had been made seriously physically ill by her medications).

So, I ended up campaigning for her release, and working with her and her legal team to secure her freedom. We attended two tribunals where her case was reviewed. It was impossible not to see these tribunals as kangaroo courts – the panel went through the motions of listening to our case but as soon as we had finished they simply asked the psychiatrists what to do – and the psychiatrists wanted to keep her detained, despite the fact that none of their treatments had done any good.

After the second tribunal I confronted one of the psychiatrists and – after quite a row – he told me to butt out because it was he and only he who would carry the can if she hurt anyone. And that was it – the only reason she was still incarcerated after nearly 3 years was this doctor's fear of being held responsible if she did anything bad once released.

After this, things got worse for me. It didn't help that the doctor in question was working in the same department in the Medical School where I was lecturing, and I soon found myself receiving couriered threats of dismissal from my post for acting 'against the university's interests'.

But – I am proud to say – I carried on regardless. On the psychiatrist's logic she would never be released – she was a young woman with a life to live and I was not going to stand by and watch it disappear fruitlessly. We appealed to the tribunal, we recruited more help still, and in the end we won – she was grudgingly released and as far as I know was never again an involuntary patient, nor did she ever hurt anyone.

Had I not been aware that ethics pervades everything I might not have seen her case as an ethical issue for me.

Ethics and health workers

Most health workers still see only the tip of the iceberg. Unfortunately:

1 Even now many receive very limited, or even no formal training in ethical reasoning, even though their daily work involves direct and often crucial intervention in other people's lives.

Figure 25 Both everyday and technical ethics should be applied to the whole iceberg

2 If they do get training in ethics it is almost always misconceived – typically lecturers in medical ethics talk about 'principles' as if they are laws, and encourage students to behave according to the lecturer's own moral preferences. Many books on ethics speak in a language and manner that most health workers find alien (numerous examples of such books can be found on library shelves at the Dewey classifications 170–174 or Library of Congress reference BJ). Although health work throws up interesting cases by the hour, the examples given to illustrate moral theory in these books are frequently artificial and hypothetical. And if real cases are used – as is the fashion in contemporary 'bioethics' – they are almost always dramatic – so, equally if not more misleading than the imaginary ones.
3 Health workers have urgent practical jobs which allow them little time to pause for thought. Furthermore, there is little provision within traditional health services for classes and discussion groups to enable health workers to reflect more deeply on the ethics of their practice.

Summary

It was argued in **Chapter One** that there is an intellectual crisis in health care, and that its future form depends both upon which theories of health come to dominate and how present health workers choose to intervene in their clients' lives. It was contended that the most desirable future – the best new paradigm – will come into being once health workers better understand the nature of ethics and its necessary relationship with work for health.

Further points and clarifications have been made in **Chapter Two:**

Summary (Continued)

1 Work for health is a moral endeavour because work for health can release more or less human potential. While it is impossible to say definitively that work for health is a particular, specific type of moral endeavour, it is vital to remember that health work is always a moral endeavour of some kind – health care is never ever a matter of evidence alone.

2 Ethics is a complex field, not merely a means of deciding between clear-cut rights and wrongs. Ultimately ethics is a matter of personal deliberation.

3 Enlightening distinctions can be made between everyday ethics and technical ethics, and between dramatic ethics, persisting ethics and ethics in the general sense.

4 Technical ethics can be divided into different aspects. Ethics as deliberation is the aspect preferred in this book since it emphasises both process and aim and is based on the notion of ethics in the general sense.

Problems of Practice

Introduction

Theoretically informed, practical solutions to the question: 'what ought to be done in health care's name?' require systematic, humane analysis. To arrive consistently at high quality answers takes practice. But given an understanding of ethical reasoning and how to do it, health workers' ethical skills can be greatly improved by regular exercise on real world cases.

The case studies and questions set out in this chapter offer an initial workout. Doing them is unlikely to turn practitioners into first class ethical analysts overnight, but the exercises should be attempted at this stage of the book nonetheless, in order to show (if further proof be needed) that some form of ethical reflection is indispensable in health work.

Each exercise should be revisited with the aid of the Ethical Grid (see **Chapter Nine**) once this instrument has been studied. Readers are also strongly encouraged to register on the free, public Values Exchange (www.values-exchange.com) to share their reflections with, and learn from, other users of the decision-making tools introduced in this book.

At the time of writing the Values Exchange was listing several practice cases, including these four:

Case ED-33 – Public Health Ethics - Closes Dec 26, 2007

Informal Consultation - Alcohol »

The Nuffield Council on Bioethics is running a public consultation on Ethical Issues in Public Health. The effects of excessive consumption of alcohol on the health of individuals and society are well-known - why are public health measures lagging behind those for tobacco?

read more

It is proposed that alcohol will be legislated against with the same force as tobacco

Sign-in to record your views »

Case H-32 – Best interests? - Closes Dec 26, 2007

Should the operation go ahead? »

Pat has a learning disability. She needs an operation to remove an ovarian cyst. If left untreated the cyst will cause renal failure. Pat vigorously resists having a needle inserted to deliver the necessary anaesthetic.

read more

It is proposed that the treatment is in the patient's best interests

Sign-in to record your views »

Case H-30 – Power over life and death - Closes Dec 26, 2007

Should Baby MB's life be prolonged? »

The family of Baby MB are fighting a hospital's bid for permission to withdraw ventilation from the 17-month-old. Doctors say it would be better to let him die as his life is "intolerable". But the child's father says no-one but God has the right to decide if the baby should live or die.

read more

It is proposed that ventilation will continue indefinitely

Sign-in to record your views »

Case ED-28 – Health Priorities - Closes Dec 26, 2007

Should Herceptin be offered on the NHS? »

A breast cancer patient should have the drug Herceptin, according to a landmark ruling from the Court of Appeal on April 12th. Ann Marie Rogers successfully appealed an earlier High Court decision upholding Swindon Primary Care Trust's refusal to fund Herceptin.

read more

It is proposed that Herceptin should be offered on the NHS to everyone who needs it

Sign-in to record your views »

Figure 26 Screenshot of some free-to-public Values Exchange, December 2007 (www.values-exchange. com)

Given that a major theme of this book is that current health work is limited by over-emphasis on the elimination and prevention of disease and illness, it might appear strange that all 15 case studies have to do with disease or illness in some way. However, medical work against disease and illness is conventionally a part of work for health and will remain so (I merely hope that focusing on current health work practice – and what is missing from it – may accelerate the paradigm change a little).

None of the case studies has an obviously right answer. There are always alternative courses of action – often several – open to the participants in each study. Any of them require justification. Why this solution and not another one?

When attempting to tackle each problem it will be productive for any interested reader to write down the course of action she would take or advise, together with her reasons and any criticisms of rejected options. Alternatively she might simply write down her feelings and intuitions about the cases. It may be enlightening for her to consider later, when the nature of ethics and the reasoning behind various ethical theories has been explained in more detail, whether her understanding of her proposals has been enlarged.

The case studies

Every case study raises an assortment of issues, not all of which will be immediately apparent. Tasks are suggested at the foot of each study for those readers who wish to begin to explore the moral issues independently or in groups.

Those readers who would like to explore a case from this book on the Values Exchange are invited to browse to www.values-exchange.com and tackle **Case H-35: The truth, the whole truth . . .** (this case is based upon Case 7 in this book):

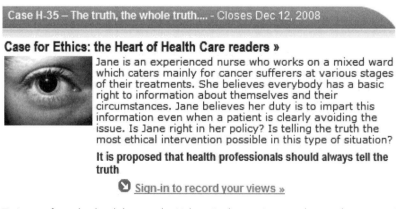

Figure 27 A case from this book live on the Values Exchange (www.values-exchange.com)

1 Teaching or caring: Michael and Caroline

Michael is a health visitor, devoted to his profession. He feels it allows him to do professionally what he would wish to do voluntarily anyway. He believes passionately that the primary reason for any person's existence is to help others.

A sensitive man who empathises naturally with nearly everyone he meets, Michael lives to care. He has the gift of seeing life as other people see it. He can shift easily into the attitudes of those he looks after. Michael often says that the secret of good health visiting is 'to be able to step temporarily into the other person's shoes'. The trouble – if indeed it is a trouble – is that some of his many friends worry that sometimes Michael's temporary becomes a little too permanent.

The seeds of this situation were sown during Michael's time as a student health visitor. An incident which happened at the end of his training upset him profoundly, so much so that he was unable to articulate fully all the aspects that distressed him. As part of his fieldwork experience Michael was assigned an elderly lady to visit once a month, between October and June. Caroline was 79, a widow, rather frail but still able to cook and clean. She had a home help twice a week. She did not suffer from any disease as far as anyone knew, and the only medication she needed was a good-sized tumbler of neat whisky every evening.

Caroline could reflect on a rich life. She had married twice, once to a journalist and then – several years after her divorce – to a successful businessman. She had been able to travel widely with both her husbands, meeting an enormous variety of people on the way, and had written about her experiences in two books. Her problem now was loneliness. Her husband had died 3 years before, and she still missed him desperately.

Michael did not see his health visiting role from a medical perspective. Indeed, his brief was simply to observe and support Caroline. He did not consider himself primarily a nurse (he was basically supposed to make sure Caroline did not suffer physical illness and injury) even though he accepts this is an important role for health visitors in many contexts. Rather Michael felt his role was to befriend the widow, to help her see the past with fondness instead of regret and longing, to help her focus on the talents and possibilities that still remained open to her, and to encourage her to share herself with other people.

Over the months Michael and Caroline became friends, despite the 45 year age gap. Though the process had been slow, Caroline had begun to think about what she could do now rather than what she had done in the past. As for Michael, he was pleased with what he was achieving with Caroline, and he too had developed. Caroline had built up a hard edge, a cynicism, during her dealings with people in journalism and business. Her stories, her accounts of her decisions and of the politics of life, saddened the committed altruist, but he recognised a certain truth in what she was saying, a necessity about what she had done. Michael was benefiting too.

Then, for reasons his superior refused to outline, Michael was assigned a different case load when he qualified, even though he was still operating the same 'patch' as before. Michael explained that he believed he was doing useful work with Caroline, and what was more he was enjoying it and thought it right to continue. But all his supervisor would say was that the old lady's circumstances did not merit the services of a busy health visitor. She was, she had to say, useful only as part of the 'learning experience'. Michael said that in that case he would continue to visit Caroline in a private capacity, but his supervisor replied curtly that this would not be advisable. It would be unprofessional behaviour.

Exercise

Write out the key issues as they occur to you.

State your approval or disapproval of any of the interventions made in this study.

Suggest ways in which things could be done differently (by any of the characters), in order to achieve a higher degree of morality.

Explain what you take 'higher degree of morality' to mean – in other words, spell out your current ethical commitment.

As far as you can, justify your opinions and suggestions.

(Remember that once you have grasped the Ethical Grid you can revisit this case.)

2 Telling the truth?

Two health education officers, Barbara and Kim, have been instructed to launch a campaign to improve local people's diets. They work in a small department managed by a district health education officer. The department is based in an inner-city area in the north-west of England, and the two officers are familiar with its high unemployment, avoidable disease and general deprivation. Both Barbara and Kim are Social Science graduates, well-equipped to research their subject area.

The District Medical Officer, who manages the District Health Education Advisor and makes policy decisions, has instructed that the campaign must be based solely on the guidelines presented in a recently published Health Authority booklet.

Barbara and Kim consider what to do. Kim decides almost immediately that she must, as a responsible and professional health education officer, carry out her orders to the letter. But Barbara has several worries.

First, she has found out that the costs of publishing the booklet were born equally by the official Health Education body and the butter industry. Second, Barbara has come to the conclusion that although the booklet is sumptuously produced – colourful, graphic and glossy – it is very hard to read. In fact it is far from clear what the practical advice is. Barbara wonders whether it is possible the information has been presented in this way deliberately in order to confuse, so that people stick with their present habits. She cannot be sure of the intentions of the writers and artists, but is worried about the effects the booklet might have. Third, from her research she has learnt that some of the information (in this case especially about fats) is significantly incomplete, to the extent that a biased picture appears to have been presented. Fourth, Barbara is not at all sure that the information and advice – the 'nutrition facts' – given in the booklet are necessarily the truth. Much of it seems to be opinion rather than certainty. To expound opinion in the guise of fact seems to Barbara to be propaganda, and she does not want to be involved in a brainwashing exercise.

Barbara has spent time exploring the history of nutrition research and advice and realises that much depends upon the fashions of the time, the social trends of a particular era, the types of foods available and the amount of money people have to spend on food. She has also read alternative theories to those presented in the booklet, and knows that informed commentators dispute several of the booklet's claims. Furthermore, when the social nature of her assigned 'patch' is taken into account it is questionable whether or not the campaign will be effective. It could turn out to be a waste of time and money. People living in nearby tower blocks, in damp, noisy, crowded conditions, unable to find work and under considerable

2 Telling the truth?   (Continued)

pressure from life's iniquitous burdens are unlikely to change the comforting habits of a lifetime because of glossy advice delivered by a pair of reasonably well-off, middle-class health education officers.

Barbara explains her worries and findings to Kim, who listens and understands Barbara's point of view, but nonetheless insists on doing her duty as a health education officer working for the health service. She can, she says, hardly do anything other than defer to the opinion of a qualified medic.

Exercise

Write out the key issues as they occur to you.

In your opinion, which of the health education officers is attempting to intervene with the highest degree of morality?

Explain what you take 'higher degree of morality' to mean – in other words, spell out your current ethical commitment.

What should Barbara do? How might she behave in this situation in order to achieve the highest degree of morality as she understands it? How do you think Barbara understands this phrase?

As far as you can, justify your opinions and suggestions.

3 To immunise or not?

Diane is a health visitor employed by a Health Authority responsible for the health of 5 million citizens. The Authority is chaired by an ambitious man, and has an uncompromising policy on immunisation and vaccination. The chairman is determined that his district will return the best vaccination figures in the country. He sees the task as a sales campaign and each employee as an agent for the policy – as a sales representative, in other words. An aggressive policy is also strongly advocated by the Specialist in Community Medicine (Child Health). Various pressures have been brought to bear on all local general practitioners to ensure they are as effective as possible in the campaign, but it is the health visitors who are seen as the main 'message-bearers' since it is possible for them to exert direct pressure on clients – on mothers whose children are due for immunisation. Such phrases as: 'go on, its the right thing to do', 'you really must agree, all the other Mums have', 'its much safer than not vaccinating', 'I've had all mine done' and 'its only fair on the child, you know' can be very powerful when said by professionals to women uncertain what to do, lack the means to research the pros and cons for themselves and want the best for their children.

The Authority's target is a straightforward 100% uptake for all those who show no contra-indications. The main thrust of the present campaign is set against whooping cough. The health visitors have been instructed to convince every parent or guardian of each child visited that the vaccination is *definitely* in the interest of each child. But Diane has doubts. She has researched the subject and, against the current tide of opinion, has arrived at the view that the risks of immunisation outweigh the benefits[61,62] and that this is what the campaign ought to be saying, while at the same time offering the service to those who wish it. Diane knows

(continued)

3 To immunise or not? (Continued)

that she would not choose to have her child vaccinated, and so she cannot honestly advocate vaccination.

Diane decides first that she is not prepared to run the risk of directly inflicting injury upon another human being. She would prefer instead to make sure that each child is fit, well-housed and well-nourished, and so better able to cope with whooping cough if it strikes. Second, Diane is opposed to a high-pressure sales campaign because she is not prepared to frighten another person unnecessarily, or to inflict stress and guilt upon someone who refuses to cooperate.

Diane's problem is that as a professional working for the State she has a contractual duty to follow the instructions she has been given. If she fails to do so she must accept possible dismissal, and even legal action, if a parent can show that Diane gave false or misleading information. Yet as an individual in her own right, as a person with opinions she feels she can justify, Diane believes she should not obey the Health Authority's command. She believes the campaign is deceitful and probably dangerous, and that less overall benefit will result from it than her pre-ferred policy.

Diane thinks the true hub of the issue is not actually to do with whether it is better to immunise or not. The evidence for and against is uncertain, and there are risks associated with vaccination that no one can honestly deny. Given this uncertainty Diane perceives that what is at stake is how people treat others. She is, she believes, being asked to lie, to coerce and to treat adults as if they are children who can cope only with simplicities and one side of the story. She does not wish to be party to what she regards as a mass insult against the local people, even one genuinely intended to be for the good of the population as a whole. What is good is arguable, and Diane thinks there are a number of possible candidates for the title 'supreme good' in this case. Among these are the notions of respect for fellow persons, and regarding and treating other people as intellectually valuable and autonomous, or potentially autonomous. Diane casts these goods, on this occasion, above the good of possibly preventing physical harm.

Diane also takes into account the fact that middle-class children are vaccinated to raise herd immunity, although those children are not in personal need of it.[62] This is never explained to their parents for fear they might refuse, even though it would be far more respectful and honest for the advocates of childhood immunisation to ask them to consider allowing the vaccinations for the sake of others.

Exercise

In this case study it is possible to focus attention on Diane alone, which is why her beliefs have been explained in detail. What should she do to achieve the highest moral intervention in this case? Before listing options and trying to justify them it is important to note that Diane appears to have some stark choices, and faces a difficult decision.

What do you think? Should Diane:

- Obey the rules as behoves a professional? If you think she should obey these rules against her better judgement, where should a health worker draw the line and disobey? Do you, for instance, think professionals should obey *any* rule that is (explicitly or implicitly) part of their job description? Should they lie? Steal? Coerce? Kill?
- Resign or be sacked? In either case she could be sure that someone else would come along and follow the rules in her stead.
- Somehow manipulate the system to achieve the end she believes to be the most moral, while remaining in the job?

4 Sponsorship and hidden motives

Professor O'Brien is Head of a Department of Community Medicine, and would like his department to be involved in as many research projects beneficial to the community as possible. The
professor also wishes to employ as many research staff as he can because he well appreciates
that it is becoming increasingly difficult for young academics to find posts at plausible universities. Dr O'Brien has an idea for a research project to discover the reasons why there is a relatively
low use of the medical and health facilities, including a health centre and a well-women's centre,
in one part of the city. The area in question is the poorest in the district, and has the highest
levels of unemployment and single-parent families, so the uptake rate is predictably low.
However, the precise reasons for the under-use of the facilities are not known. Considering that
the local population suffers a disproportionately high level of disease and illness it seems
unquestionably important to understand more about why the people act as they do.

It is here that the controversy begins. Professor O'Brien has exhausted his research budget
so he makes it known to potential sponsors and research bodies that he wishes to embark on
a 2-year project, employing at least one research fellow. Unfortunately for the professor, none
of the usual sources of funds wishes or is able to help. However, out of the blue there comes
an offer of sponsorship from a famous tobacco company. The company tells Professor O'Brien
that it hopes to fund worthwhile health research throughout the country and is pleased to say
that this is one of its first offers: it is prepared, up to a certain financial limit, to fund for 3 years
a community project of Dr O'Brien's choosing.

The nature of the problem could hardly be more clear: should Professor O'Brien accept
sponsorship from a company that trades in a commodity known to cause disease and illness?

Exercise

Write out the key issues as they occur to you.

State your approval or disapproval of the actions made in this study so far.

Explain what you think Professor O'Brien should do. How can he achieve the highest degree
of morality in these circumstances?

Explain what you take 'higher degree of morality' to mean – in other words, spell out your
current ethical commitment.

As far as you can, justify both your theoretical position and your practical proposals.

5 Tragic choices: The nurse practitioner's dilemma

Unlike most of these case studies, in which a range of alternatives are possible, this dilemma
is at the sharp end of moral philosophy – dramatic ethics. It sits at the tip of the iceberg,
posing the type of predicament[63] typically relished by moral philosophers, where the decision-
maker is faced with two choices – both of which she has a *prima facie* duty to make – but
can choose only one. Whatever she decides there will be a high price to pay.

The French philosopher Jean-Paul Sartre gave this example of a tragic choice: in the Second
World War a young man has to choose between leaving home to fight with the French Resistance, or staying to protect and look after his frail mother, who would have to live alone if
he were to leave. What, if he is to be moral, is the young man to do?

There are no more 'tragic choice' case studies in this book because such cases are exceptional.
They are simply not the everyday experience of health workers. Occasionally health workers

(Continued)

5 Tragic choices: The nurse practitioner's dilemma (Continued)

will be faced with them, so it is useful to have some experience of their analysis. However, it is essential to remember that there are no neutral human interventions: dramatic ethical dilemmas are merely the most easily seen.

Nurse practitioners work from some health centres in the UK, USA and other developed nations. Patients are sometimes able to consult them as an alternative to seeing a doctor. Nurse practitioners can recommend some treatments and will refer patients on where necessary.

Sandra is a pioneering nurse practitioner who has quickly built up a list of patients who find it easier to deal with her than the doctors. Her clinician partners do not resent this since they recognise the benefits of Sandra's presence, to themselves and the patients.

Sandra is about to attend a seminal national meeting in which a proposal to extend the nurse practitioner programme to all parts of the country will be either agreed or rejected. As an articulate pioneer her attendance is crucial. It could mean the difference between nurse practitioners becoming a recognised part of health services or remaining on the periphery of official health care for the foreseeable future.

As Sandra is about to leave for the meeting the receptionist rushes to tell her that one of her patients is on the phone, threatening to commit suicide and insisting on seeing her. Sandra knows the patient is highly strung and sensitive, and knows too that she is probably the only one who will be able to help. She knows she could very well save the distraught woman's life.

Her dilemma is crystal clear: should she stay to help her patient, or should she go to the meeting to help ensure that more nurse practitioners become available to aid many more people, and possibly save many more lives?

Exercise

Write out the key issues as they occur to you.

Explain which of the options open to Sandra you favour.

Explain why you think your preference would achieve the higher degree of morality. To stay or to go. Both options might be justified. As you try to substantiate your choice take careful note of the reasons you give – these are part of your so far unanalysed moral position. Later in the book, once you have the advantage of the Ethical Grid, you will be able to test out the strength of these thoughts.

6 Is coercion acceptable?: The forthright district nurse

Coercion is constraining or compelling a person into thinking or doing something she would not otherwise have done. Is it ever right to coerce a person, either for that person's own good or for the good of society? This question inevitably raises others. For example, is coercion *always* undesirable? Can coercion ever be justified, and if so on what ground? What factors should be taken into consideration before the imposition of a medically defined 'good' on another person? Is it enough that the coercer possesses knowledge impossible or undesirable to transmit to the coerced? Or does another's lack of knowledge place other obligations on the person with superior information?

6 Is coercion acceptable?: The forthright district nurse (Continued)

Anne is a district nurse with strong views against smoking. Her position has become dog-matic over the last 6 months as a result of her work with two families whose lives have been thrown into temporary chaos by the death from lung cancer of one member of each (in one case the mother and in the other the father). Coincidentally, both deceased used to smoke over 30 cigarettes a day and had done so consistently for many years. In Anne's opinion there is simply no question that both deaths were directly attributable to their habits. Both people would still be alive, in all probability for 20 or so more years, if they had not smoked.

Anne has now come up with a strategy to deal with smoking problems in other families. She regards smoking as a simple evil which ought to be totally stamped out. She cannot see that smoking has any benefits at all, and nor does she allow any distinction between types of smoker, on any ground. Of course, more sophisticated views than Anne's are pos-sible. For example, one might distinguish between those whose habit harms no one else and those who are smoking in homes shared by young families; or one might distinguish between those smoking who wish to give up and those who believe smoking is helpful to them in some way. Perhaps they are very nervous and smoking helps them relax, and they consider the side-effects of smoking a price worth paying for this relaxation. But Anne accepts no such prevarication. Her aim is to stop the habit, whatever the reasons people have for smoking.

Her strategy has five stages:

1 She always makes it clear that on no account is smoking permitted during her visit to a home.
2 Anne states emphatically that there is absolutely no doubt that smoking causes cancer.
3 Anne offers, and always leaves anyway, anti-smoking pamphlets and information about why it is stupid to smoke.
4 Anne deliberately changes her attitude from friendliness to hostility when she knows one of her clients is continuing to smoke despite her advice.
5 If her patient continues to refuse to cooperate then Anne's strategy is the severest she can apply. For a time Anne continues to provide the minimum treatment necessary for the condi-tion, but she makes it clear that she could do more, and will – just so long as the patient gives up. If even this fails to produce the desired result Ann refuses treatment until the smoker gives up.

Exercise

Write out the key issues as they occur to you.
State your approval or disapproval of the various parts of Anne's strategy, and of the strategy in total.
Suggest ways (if you think there are any) in which the degree of morality of Anne's anti-smoking intervention could be increased.
Justify your opinions and suggestions as vigorously as you can.
(Note: it is important to consider legal issues in this case.)

7 Death and the truth

Jane is an experienced nurse who works on a mixed ward which caters mainly for cancer sufferers at various stages of their treatments. Jane is a Catholic and very single-minded about telling the truth. She believes everybody has a basic right to information about themselves and their circumstances, especially when they are in hospital. And when the relevant information is that they will soon be dead Jane believes she has an absolute duty to tell this to her patients. Not only does she feel obliged to do so, but she argues that certain benefits follow too. Once they know the truth patients are able to prepare themselves, their relatives and their friends – and to make their peace with God. Jane believes her duty is to impart this information even when a patient is clearly avoiding the issue, even when the relatives ask that the patient not be told and even if the medical judgement is that the knowledge would cause psychological damage.

Is Jane right in her policy? Is telling the truth the most ethical intervention possible in this type of situation?

Exercise

Write out the key issues as they occur to you.
State your approval or disapproval of Jane's policy.
Suggest alternative policies for intervention which would create a higher degree of morality
  in this context.
Try to justify your opinions and suggestions.
Now have a go at this case on the Values Exchange (www.values-exchange.com).

8 Is all drug education health education?

Kathy is a thoughtful and conscientious health education officer. Her manager has decided that Kathy will be responsible for the local campaign against 'drug misuse', but Kathy is of the view that some of this material is misleading. Some is quite clearly designed to shock. For example, there are several graphic posters that predict death, physical disability or a zombie-like existence as an inevitable consequence of using illicit drugs. Furthermore, at least as it appears to Kathy, some of the campaign material sets out to create such myths as cannabis smoking will lead inevitably to smoking or injecting heroin; experimenting with heroin means instant dependency for the user; illegal drugs are the only truly dangerous drugs; all illegal drugs are equally liable to create dependency; and the use of drugs means that the user will eventually be unable to hold down work, or be unable to have a social life with people who do not use drugs. Yet further, the information Kathy has been asked to distribute pays insufficient attention, in her opinion, to the fact that a major cause of dependency arises from addiction to prescribed drugs such as tranquillisers (which can create a dependency from which it is unpleasant and difficult to withdraw).[64]

Kathy hates the thought that a person's major interest in life is finding ways to escape from it. She is strongly in favour of preventing dependency on drugs and of offering alternative means for people to find life worthwhile, yet she is equally earnestly opposed to deception and gross exaggeration of the truth, whatever the motivation of the person who seeks to deceive.

8 Is all drug education health education? (Continued)

Kathy is also increasingly disturbed that, directly and explicitly, she has become an agent for the government. She doesn't think this is necessarily a bad thing but, because she is losing control over what she does, she thinks she has cause for concern.

Kathy has outlined her apprehension to the District Health Education Advisor, who referred her to the District Medical Officer, who told her kindly that she must do as she is told by her superiors. This means, in practice, that Kathy is obliged by her employer to ensure that the posters are placed in libraries and other public places, and that Kathy faces a very tricky decision over the content of her lectures to groups of teenagers. She is supposed to follow the official line but knows (she is only 24) that this strategy will be ineffective – even counter-productive with such groups, many of whom will have tried, and if not will almost certainly know people who have tried, illegal drugs and not experienced the tales of horror she has been told to frighten them with. She also has to deal with a similar problem – which she sees ultimately as a question of personal integrity – as she decides on the content of a talk to a group of parents, many of whom will expect to have the government hyperbole confirmed.

Exercise

Write out the key issues as they occur to you.

Explain how Kathy might act in order to create the highest degree of morality, and offer the strongest defence of this policy that you can.

Explain what you take 'higher degree of morality' to mean – in other words, spell out your current ethical commitment.

How would you summarise Kathy's ethical commitment (her Ethics B – see the **Introduction to the Second Edition**).

9 Rationing health services

It's just after midnight. The doors of the A&E department burst open as a semi-conscious man is dragged through by two supporters. One of them half collapses into a chair, hauling his burden with him. The other approaches the reception desk.

'Arapeta's crook, eh?'

'Pardon?' enquires the receptionist. 'What did you say?'

'My bro man, he's shot. We've been on the piss eh, but he can take it man. He don't usually get like this, eh.'

The receptionist looks across the room. She sees an obviously overweight man, in his late thirties or thereabouts, of Pacific Island descent, with swollen features, having difficulty breathing.

'How long has Arapeta been this way?'

'He's not been good for a while eh, a few months, eh bro?' he enquires of the other helper, who nods.

'I think he should see the triage nurse straight away, will you wait just a minute?'

The nurse arrives, briefly examines the patient, calls the doctor, and Arapeta is wheeled away from the reception area.

(Continued)

9 Rationing health services (Continued)

Two days later, after numerous tests, Arapeta is told he has advanced renal failure, in addition to his diabetes. He needs a transplant and in the meantime could benefit from dialysis, but unfortunately this service is not currently available.

What Arapeta and his friends do not know is that the consultants, managers and hospital lawyers have been involved in hot debate about whether or not to dialyse Arapeta. The majority verdict was that dialysis should not be offered (though a unit is available) because resources are limited, and it is very likely that more 'deserving candidates' will soon present.

The problem is that Arapeta is not a social asset (at least he is not as most of the decision-makers see it). He is already a diabetic, he has not had a job for years, drinks heavily and has no dependants. To treat him would, at least as one of the consultants put it, 'be an irresponsible waste of taxpayer's money'.

Without treatment Arapeta will die, and he and his friends are duly informed of this.

Exercise

Write out the key issues as they occur to you. If you need, you may add any further information necessary to allow a full deliberation. (Is there an explicit policy on dialysis? Has the public been involved? Do black people receive dialysis on an equal basis with whites? Do a greater proportion of black people need dialysis?)

What are the central moral considerations in this situation?

Do you think the decision-makers' choice has achieved the highest degree of morality?

Explain what you take 'higher degree of morality' to mean – in other words, spell out your current ethical commitment.

What could be done differently? What else should be done?

As far as you can, offer a justification and defence of your views.

10 Mental illness

It was a beautiful blue midwinter's day, so radiantly sunny it was hard for Brian Wilson to imagine how anyone could be depressed during it. Yet as a senior psychiatrist in an over-stretched and under-funded health service he was ruefully aware that even the most glorious day has only fleeting remedial power.

Dr Wilson parked outside a sparkling white villa, walked briskly through a tidy front garden, and knocked on the stained glass door. It was opened by a tall woman, in her mid-thirties, dressed in a white singlet and shorts.

'Come in Brian, please.' She turned quickly and walked along the hall, her long blonde hair catching shafts of sunlight.

'How is he, Sarah?' She stopped, and looked straight at him.

'You'll see for yourself in a minute. It's got worse now. They're trying to get rid of him.'

'Who are?'

'His partners. They sent him a letter today telling him he's in breach of contract. They want him to pack his bags within 2 days. I've been on to Ken and he's going to look into it for me. Can they do this do you think?'

10 Mental illness (Continued)

Wilson had known Paul and Sarah for several years, mostly personally but now profession-ally, and saw immediately what had happened. Paul was a GP. A couple of years previously he went into partnership with three others in a local practice, and had been doing well. About 9 months ago Paul had become withdrawn and rather depressed, and for the last few weeks had experienced strange thoughts and had been behaving increasingly oddly.

Two weeks ago, with uncanny bad luck, a snatch of his behaviour was caught on film and received national TV exposure for several days. A new casino had just opened, and for some reason Paul went to the opening ceremony (a lavish event, closed to the general public). He interrupted proceedings with shouts and screams: 'parasites', 'leeches', 'capitalist dogs', 'this is sin – all are sinners' and other slogans, more colourful still. The footage was shown every time 'protestors to the casino' were mentioned on the news, though in truth Paul was the only 'activist' there. It was gruesome publicity for the GP partnership, and had obviously prompted Paul's colleagues to move to banish him.

'How nice of them. Just what you'd expect from a caring profession', thought Brian, as he entered the comfortable living room. Paul was sitting in an easy chair, his chin on his chest in unwanted sleep.

'Paul, Paul, how are you?'

Paul shook himself, and with difficulty raised his head and opened his eyes.

'I'm OK. Just tired. This stuff is knocking me out.'

'I think we should change the medication, would that be alright?'

'Yes, sure. I've got to make calls you know.'

'What calls, Paul? Ones to your practice? That letter's bad news mate. Can I do anything?'

'You know Sarah's pregnant again don't you?' Wilson did know. In fact he was as concerned for Sarah and the other three children as he was for Paul. Sarah was superficially collected, and the pleasant house and uplifting weather imbued the situation with misleading optimism. But when she mentioned the letter her stress had been obvious. She badly needed respite from this mess.

Paul continued. 'Oh yes. That's no problem. It's time I sacked *them*. I have to arrange the concert you see.'

'I thought you were to have the concert last week', Dr Wilson said.

'Oh, yeah, but Kiri couldn't make it. She called and apologised. I said it was OK – sure I can call on a lot of help from around the globe – but I want you Kiri. You owe it to New Zealand.'

'So the concert's still on then?'

'Of course, we're going to have it when we have the regatta down the hill. Michael and Macca are cool about it.'

'Paul, you know there isn't any concert. You know there isn't. Don't go on about it again, please', Sarah intervened firmly.

'No. OK. I know it didn't work out last time but I mean I have influence and it will be good. I know it will be good now.'

Brian changed the subject. 'What were you doing at the casino?'

Paul laughed. 'Ha, I shouldn't have gone there should I? Not a good look.'

An image of Paul, kicking, yelling and holding fiercely onto the side of a descending escala-tor while burly bouncers tried to lever him off it, hung in the doctor's mind.

'No. It wasn't. I'm going to call TV Ten and tell them not to run the clip anymore. OK?'

Sarah said, 'That would be great if you could, Brian'.

'And in the meantime', Wilson had more gravity now, 'what do you think about being admitted for a few days? I want to get the meds right. And you need the rest, don't you?'

(Continued)

10 Mental illness (Continued)

'What about the concert?'

'There isn't really a concert Paul. It's a grandiose idea, you know.'

'Yes . . . No, I have arranged it and I can't cancel it now. I can't just call Michael Jackson and Paul McCartney and cancel out of the blue . . .'

'You've spoken to them before?'

'Yes. Mostly it is the agent I deal with but don't underestimate what I can do . . .' Paul stopped quite suddenly, and went to sleep again.

'Sarah, we need to get this sorted out. Do you want me to get him a bed?'

'He doesn't want to go to hospital. Does he have to?'

'He may have to, but it would be better if you got him to agree.'

Exercise

As far as you can, list the main issues as they occur to you.
Dr Wilson has at least four options available:

1 To do nothing further.
2 To change Paul's medication and continue to monitor him at home.
3 To persuade him to admit himself to a psychiatric hospital.
4 To admit him, without his agreement, to a psychiatric hospital.

Which of these options do you think will create the highest degree of morality in this difficult situation? Explain what you take 'higher degree of morality' to mean.

Can you suggest an alternative policy or policies that would create the highest degree of morality?

Try to justify your opinions and proposals.

11 Doctors and nurses

Mary has been a nurse for 27 years, and knows how to handle herself in tense circumstances. This time though, she is not sure how to act for the best.

For the last few weeks she has noticed that Dr Jones, a doctor just into his thirties, has been giving unusually high doses of morphine and other painkillers to terminally ill geriatric patients. From what she knows of him she doesn't believe he is doing anything sinister – she doesn't think he is intending to kill them – but neither does she think he is acting in their best interests. In Mary's opinion the old people are over-sedated. They spend their days asleep or sitting by themselves communicating little, if at all. And this, she thinks, is pointless.

Mary spoke to Dr Jones about the dosage, but the conversation didn't go well. The doctor was instantly defensive, and let Mary know right away that: 'It is none of your business, OK?' Despite her experience, she riled at this, and told him straight that it was, and that he ought to think very carefully about what he was doing. Dr Jones interpreted this as a threat (which it was, partly), said he wasn't going to stand for that, and told Mary to get out of 'his ward'. Angry and upset, Mary left.

And now she doesn't know what to do.

Exercise

Describe the key issues in this case. What are the main ethical pressures, do you think?
How can Mary act so as to achieve the highest degree of morality?
Why does your suggestion achieve the highest degree of morality?
Explain what you take 'higher degree of morality' to mean – in other words, spell out your
   current ethical commitment.

12 Health in a bottle?

For 6 months Pharmaceutical Industries Ltd. (PIL) has been providing a legally registered but
unsubsidised drug (EAZE) free of charge to 100 chronically ill patients. Most are young –
below 30 – and all suffer from a degenerative and incurable lung disorder. EAZE is designed
to relieve pain and breathlessness, has done so significantly in 34 cases, moderately in 27 and
has had no effect in the rest. Some of the most fortunate group feel so much better that they
have returned to work.

This week PIL has written to each patient's doctor to inform them that EAZE is no longer
to be offered compassionately. The physicians have called a patients' meeting, which is now
underway.

◆

A young man, with long yellow hair and goatee beard, is standing, his face reddening as he
tries to keep his composure.

'How can they do this to us? This drug has changed my life. I had nothing to look forward
too but now I can drive and I've got a part-time job at the college. If they take EAZE away
I'll lose it – shit, I'll lose it all.'

There is a buzz of approval from the others, and claps from some.

'Richard', one of the doctors replies, from behind the table on the stage, 'we've been through
this a hundred times. You knew the score when you agreed to this trial. You knew you could
have the drug free for 6 months and that it would stop at that point. You agreed to it on those
terms. It was quite explicit.'

'We knew it, sure we knew it,' a painfully frail young woman stands now, in agitation. 'But
we didn't think they'd be such bastards.'

Whoops from her friends.

'We thought they wanted to help us. And we thought – this is going to work and when it
does something will change and someone will help us. Hey, we pay taxes so we're entitled
anyway. And PIL calls it compassionate supply. We thought they meant it. The drugs haven't
run out have they, so where's their compassion gone?'

There's fulsome applause at this.

'We don't make PIL's policy', says the doctors' Chair. 'Like you, we had hoped they would
extend the supply particularly because it has worked well for some of you, but they won't
have it. If you want to keep on with EAZE it's going to cost you the best part of £20,000 a
year, unless the government agrees to subsidise it, but they say they won't.

'I called William Booth today – the Junior Minister. He told me, in no uncertain terms, that
the government's drug budget is not a bottomless pit, EAZE isn't a cure, it's expensive, and
he isn't going to be blackmailed by the pharmaceutical industry.'

(Continued)

12 Health in a bottle? (Continued)

'What do you mean? PIL's been good to us. They didn't have to supply it free at all.'

'He means that PIL has used you first as a trial – to see if EAZE helps people like you – and second as a lobby group: you want EAZE and you could get it if the government chose to help pay for it, so you will put pressure on the Ministry of Health to subsidise EAZE – you're bound to.'

The yellow-haired man pulls himself to his feet again.

'Whose fault is it then? Is it our fault for wanting to get better? Sure, it must be. Is it PIL's fault – they're a business so they have to make a profit, but haven't they given us false hope? And isn't that cruel? Is it the government? They have to ration medicine, we know that, but why this one? I could accept it if I knew they'd looked as carefully at everything else they spend on, but they haven't, of course they haven't.

Where does this leave us? What am I supposed to do now? Isn't my life worth anything to anyone?'

Exercise

Distinguish the main components of this complicated case. What are the central moral concerns, as far as you can tell from the information available? Who is behaving well and who is behaving badly? Who is responsible for the health of the volunteers?

Now imagine you are the GP of four of the patients. What are you going to do? Assuming you want to achieve the highest degree of morality in this situation, how and why are you going to do it?

Explain what you take 'higher degree of morality' to mean – in other words, spell out your current ethical commitment.

13 Businessperson or care-giver?

Dr Smith has just finished a fraught call to his bank manager. The mortgage rate is up again and the doctor cannot afford the repayments on his large new house. As he switches his phone off a patient enters, and a perfectly normal consultation ensues.

It turns out the patient has a mild respiratory infection, for which the GP prescribes a broad-spectrum antibiotic. He is 98% sure it will do the trick, but he asks the patient to come back to see him in 4 days' time, so he can be certain the antibiotic is appropriate.

This, one might think, is normal and proper practice. But there is a difficulty. Dr Smith works in a country where people of reasonable means (like his patient) have to pay a fee each time they consult. This means, of course, that it is in the doctor's personal interest that the patient makes a follow-up appointment.

Exercise

Clarify the main points at issue in this case.
Assume that Dr Smith genuinely wants to work first and foremost for the health of his patient. Given this, did his intervention bring about the highest degree of morality or not? Explain your reasoning.

14 What should the lecturer do?

The second year medical students have written a petition and all 121 of them have signed it. The petition asks the Dean of the Medical School and the Vice-Chancellor of the University to act immediately to reform the medical school curriculum. Here is part of it:

'We the undersigned petition that medical students are given the same standard of education – with the same level of intellectual challenge – as all other students of this University. Though facts and skills are essential to us as future doctors we entreat that:

1 The first year programme be altered so that students do not repeat material already studied in school.
2 Pre-clinical teaching staff co-ordinate to ensure that material is not repeated.
3 A distinction is made between essential, recommended and optional learning (we presently have to spend days cramming factual material we will never use, which will soon date, or which can be easily looked up if we need it).
4 The ethics, sociology, psychology, humanities and communication components be increased as the pre-clinical load is reduced.
5 Time for student-directed learning be increased substantially.'

Dr Crossley, a young ethics lecturer, has repeatedly encouraged and supported the students in these views, and is delighted that they have written the petition. However, when the second year rep asks him to sign it, he is not sure he should. Crossley is approaching the end of a 3-year fixed term contract, has made both friends and enemies at the Medical School, and is learning that job security comes at a price. If he signs it the Dean will notice – and the Dean is shortly also to rule on whether Crossley's contract should be extended or the job advertised anew.

Exercise

Clarify the main points at issue.
Is this a health issue?
Should Crossley sign the petition?
How can Crossley best achieve the highest degree of morality?
Explain what the lecturer should do, and why he should do it.

15 A right to health care?

Dr Walker is quietly explaining to a chronically ill elderly patient that she is not going to recommend further heart surgery. An auxiliary overhears the conversation and anonymously informs the patient's son – Donald Spencer – a prominent lawyer.

Spencer makes enquiries and discovers that though the operation is risky in a woman of 81 it is clinically indicated and – if successful – could increase her mobility and extend her life. He tells his mother what has happened and what he is going to do. At this she begins to cry. She tells him that Dr Walker is a lovely woman and she doesn't want to cause her any trouble. She also says that she is not afraid to die and she hopes a younger person will benefit from the operation instead.

Donald is furious. He tells his mother that he hears the doctor speaking, not his mum. 'Dad would never forgive you if you give up now. You are being discriminated against on the ground of age. This is a human rights issue and I'm going to fight tooth and claw to get what you are entitled to.' His mother merely sighs, and sinks back on her pillow.

Her son walks purposefully from the room, in search of Dr Walker.

Exercise

As with all the exercises, add further information if you need it.

Imagine you are either Dr Walker or Donald Spencer. What are the key issues from your point of view? Why are these the most important issues? Is this basically a human rights issue as Spencer thinks, or are there more important moral considerations?

How should Dr Walker respond to Spencer's angry request to operate on his mother? At this crucial point, how should Dr Walker bring about the highest degree of morality?

Summary

This chapter has offered 15 studies of the sorts of situations that may be faced by health workers. It is hoped that the chapter will serve both as a source of teaching material and as background to the discussion contained in the remainder of this book.

Most of the case studies are not dramatic. Some may have appeared rather ordinary, perhaps even to the point where it was difficult to see how they are to do with ethics at all. But each, when analysed and thought through, raises moral questions of immense significance. All health workers – nurses, doctors, auxiliaries, chaplains, social workers, non-medical staff, consultants, managers, teachers, administrators and patients – are involved in daily interaction in the moral realm. The secret is to recognise this. Once a health worker is aware of the extent to which morality impregnates her work she can take steps to ensure that she directs her activity towards boosting morality in every situation (whatever she takes this to mean).

By using this book you can see how these situations can be dealt with by use of two printed decision-making tools (see **Chapters Eight and Nine**), by seeing the decision-making process as a series of rational fields (see the **Introduction to the Third Edition**) and by use of the Values Exchange software system (see **Chapter Eleven** and www.values-exchange.com).

The Search for Morality

Introduction

I have taken the unusual step of retaining a mistaken argument (included in the First and Second Editions) in order to show how this edition's thesis has moved on. The parts of the argument I still uphold are presented in the same font as the rest of the book. The parts I now reject are presented in this font, and the parts where I discuss the mistake are presented *like this* (see, for example, p. 66).

This chapter embarks on a search to discover clear examples of morality. This turns out to be a false hope, but a solid base for ethical practice is unearthed nevertheless.

The problem with the ambition to find 'the truly moral' is that people hold beliefs and values whose truth or falsity cannot be objectively assessed. The statement 'water boils at 100° Celsius at sea level' is testable. It can be shown to be true provided the definitions included in it, and the method of testing, are agreed. But the statement 'it is right to perform euthanasia on a patient who has repeatedly requested it' cannot be empirically tested. It may be possible to establish how many times and under what conditions the patient expressed the wish, but it is impossible to discover experimentally whether or not a health worker would be morally right to assist.

This basic difficulty is further elucidated in this chapter. Afterwards, various attempts to resolve value conflicts are discussed, and five possibilities are considered:

1 Finding some ultimate value or ordering of values.
2 Finding a set of rules.
3 Appealing to the law.
4 Settling for relativism.
5 Making an appeal to the relevant facts.

(**Note:** I now think that rational fields are the solution – see my discussion of this idea in the **Introduction to the Third Edition**.)

The question of value

Any answer one might give to the problems raised in the case studies (see **Chapter Three**) must involve some reference to values. For instance, if you feel that Kathy (the health education officer instructed to carry out a radical campaign against drug misuse – Case 8) is right in her misgivings, then though your thinking may be based on an assessment of likely consequences, at some point opinion must also have a role. Perhaps it will be thought that Kathy should have more autonomy, or that the public has a right to be informed rather than frightened, or that teenagers should be told the bare truth, or that recreational drug use is not a medical issue. The opposite point of view, perhaps that Kathy should conform to the wisdom of her more experienced superiors, or that any course of action is justified if it helps eliminate drug abuse, also rests ultimately on values. Whatever you think, you will inevitably make value judgements.

What are values?

It seems natural for us to consider some physical things more valuable than others – a motor car, for instance, usually seems more valuable (both financially and practically) than a bar of chocolate. We also tend to think of less tangible things as more or less valuable. For example, most of us consider that happiness is to be valued above misery, that life is better than death, that pain is bad, that work and creativity are to be admired, that owning property is desirable, that truth-telling is worthwhile and that trying to help friends is important.

Distinguishing values

How can different types of value be distinguished from one another? And how can this be done so that more light is thrown upon the nature of morality?

The analysis of values given here is by no means exhaustive. However, it is useful to note: (a) that different types of valuing have different ethical implications; and (b) that all valuing is done by subjects who exist within a wider culture.[10]

1 Different types of valuing have different ethical implications

If a person values a principle such as 'the truth must always be told', then her conviction can have implications for ethics in the dramatic, persisting and general senses. However, if a person holds an aesthetic value (if she values a picture or a poem, for instance) or another type of intangible value (perhaps she values a relationship) then the mere fact that she has the value does not necessarily raise dramatic or persisting ethical issues – though maintaining any value always has some bearing on ethics in the general sense (because ethics in the general sense has to do with how a person chooses to live her life, and values are necessary foundations of social behaviour).

Types of valuing

The following categories are not impervious, and overlap in significant ways. They are, however, a helpful clarification in the search for morality.

Most simply, a person can be said to have a value when he finds something – anything – valuable. More specifically:

i It is customary – at least in wealthy societies – for people to value *physical things*, such as DVD players, money and pets (either as means, ends, or both). This type of valuing (and all the other types listed below too) can be said to relate to morality in different ways, dependent upon what is meant by morality, and dependent upon which part of the 'ethics iceberg' (see **Chapter Two**) is perceived as most important at a particular time. Consider your neighbour's house, for example. If morality is merely a question of right and wrong (a form of dramatic ethics) and it is thought that certain moral rules or commandments define what is right, then valuing property will be either right or wrong depending on how you look at the world. If it is a moral rule that it is wrong to covet another person's property, and you covet your neighbour's house, then valuing that physical thing is morally wrong. If the moral rule is that coveting other people's property is good (perhaps because it may inspire greater effort on your part) then valuing that physical thing is morally right. Furthermore, if you value your house and there is no ruling about whether this is right or wrong, then valuing this physical thing is neither morally right nor wrong, according to the 'right and wrong' view of ethics. (Seen from other parts of the iceberg the question: is it moral to covet my neighbour's house? can look quite different, and is certainly more complex than the 'right and wrong' view allows.)

ii It is obviously possible to value objects – works of art and beautiful gardens, for instance – for their *aesthetic qualities*. Again, whether or not such valuing has a moral aspect depends upon what morality is said to mean.

iii Similarly, it is possible to value *intangibles*, such as friendship, introspection and creativity.

iv It is possible to value *principles*. Whether or not these should be described as moral principles depends on what they are and – again – on how morality is defined. If one values moral principles then it becomes necessary to reflect on them (to conceive of them)[8] and to arrive at judgements about whether or not they are worth holding and are consistent with other principles espoused. If a person holds principles that are in some way incoherent then it is her task – as she thinks about how she should live – to make incongruities apparent, so she might improve her personal reasoning. For example, if a person holds the principle 'all life is sacred' and is therefore absolutely opposed to vivisection, yet also believes that in order to protect national sovereignty it is fundamentally right to go to war, then he is not making sense and must decide which principle is most important, or must express a yet more fundamental principle which somehow allows him to convert 'all life is sacred' into 'some life is sacred, some of the time'.

v It is possible to value *ideologies*, such as patriotism, liberalism, fascism or communism.

2 All valuing is done by subjects within a culture

All human beings capable of intellectual reflection have values. Some of these may be innate (we seem to be biologically programmed to value our own lives and those of our offspring, for instance) but any attempt to give a comprehensive list of 'innate' values would be a ceaselessly controversial exercise.

Some values undoubtedly depend upon the culture and era in which the subject exists. For example, paid work is almost universally valued in contemporary society, but such valuing is possible only if such an institution (work for a fee) exists.[64,65] Furthermore, given the existence of something potentially valuable, people can obviously be encouraged to value it (this is what advertisers do all the time) – a phenomenon that prompts important questions about the difference between human values and morality. For instance, it is in the interests of capitalist businesses that people value paid work but – just because paid work has become a desired social norm – does this mean it is a moral activity?

Morality or value – which is basic?

It is interesting to ask which notion – human value or human morality – is basic.
   Options:

i It is possible that cultural values create all moral principles and reasoning. If this were the case morality would depend entirely on human values generated by prevailing cultural norms. Whichever values were predominant in a particular culture would be the source of that culture's moral principles. For example, if 'social stability' and 'racial purity' were fundamental values then – in that particular culture – moral principles would be specified in such a way as to perpetuate them.
ii It is possible that cultural values and morality are independent. In this case it would be possible, for example, to say with moral authority that although racial purity is valued, polices to ensure it are nevertheless unethical.
iii It is possible that cultural values and morality are partially separate and partially dependent (which is the proposal advocated in this book – and extended in the discussion of rational fields in the **Introduction to the Third Edition**).
iv It is possible that moral reasoning and moral principles create cultural values. (Note, though, that if this were the case morality would somehow have to exist beyond or before culture. And one would, therefore, expect different cultures to have identical or similar basic values.)

Consolidation

A link has been established between human value and morality, although the precise nature of this association remains at issue. In the section that follows it is shown that values are an essential part of health work. This, of course, is further evidence of the depth of health work's moral content.

Values permeate all health work

It can be tempting to think that work for health is value-free – that some endeavours are good, desired by all and therefore unequivocally moral.

For example, it can seem obvious that there can be no question that curing disease, illness and injury is good – pure and simple. Of course, in many situations – perhaps most – medical care undoubtedly ought to be described as a good thing, but it is not necessarily so. Is it, for example, unequivocally moral to attempt to cure pneumonia in a patient who is suffering the final stages of terminal cancer? Is it moral to perform a hip replacement operation on a 90-year-old suffering from senile dementia? Is it moral to allocate scarce kidney dialysis wholly on the basis of predicted life years? Is it moral to pin the broken leg of a man condemned to be executed the following day?

There are, furthermore, an indefinite number of specific choices that must made in everyday practice ('How many patients should I see each day as a GP?' 'If I don't know something or am unsure, should I admit this to the patient?'), there are choices of ward policy in hospitals ('Should we set a weight and gestation limit below which we will never attempt to resuscitate a neonate?'), and there are choices that concern the shape and organisation of health services as a whole ('Where budgets are limited, which ought to be the priority – heart transplants, cures for acne, or disease prevention campaigns?').

Careful reflection on health care practice inescapably reveals that all work for health – every last bit of it – is at some point inspired by a human value that has been chosen (implicitly or explicitly) from alternatives. And this, in turn, means that decisions about what a health service should be doing and how it should be organised are not unassailable but rest firmly on the shoulders of those who have the power to change them (a category that includes all health workers, even though most of us have little or no direct power).

Even advice to exercise is not value-free

Exercise is commonly regarded as an unquestionably good activity, something anyone who is fit enough ought to do. Some people even go so far as to argue that people have a duty to exercise, since by exercising they stand a better chance of avoiding disease and illness that might adversely affect others (family members for example) and place avoidable financial burden on the State.

A typical view that advice to exercise is value-neutral

> Everybody knows exercise is, as a matter of fact, good for you. So it must surely be true that well-intentioned advice to exercise sensibly must be a good that everyone will agree about. Advice to exercise, then, is objectively good advice, and as such must be considered value-free.

But it is not value-free. To think it is is to make the mistake of believing that what you like is what everybody else likes – or at least ought to like 'if only they knew what was good for them' – and to believe that your preference holds true universally. To make this mistake is to underrate the opinions, knowledge, attitudes and experiences of other people.

The discussion below is not intended to convey the impression that there is no practical or moral difference between exercising conscientiously and smoking 40 cigarettes a day. Obviously, not all health advice depends solely on subjective value. There are objective elements to much of it (in the above case, the effects of exercise and smoking can be measured), but there are not and cannot possibly be objectively moral elements to any of it. Even advice to exercise is biased, for the following reasons.

1 *There is no agreed definition of fitness.* One of the most commonly espoused goals of exercise is 'fitness', yet surprisingly there is no agreed definition of this term. In fact it seems impossible to offer a universal standard of fitness because people have different physiques, are of varying ages and of one of two sexes. The actual goal for individuals – the personal target they choose to call fitness – will always depend to some extent on subjective opinions about what fitness is, and about what activities they want to be fit for. A decision about whether stamina, suppleness, muscle development, or some combination of these factors is of most importance for personal fitness can be informed by detailed measurement and investigation, but must ultimately depend upon a judgement about which is desirable.

Furthermore, any person's fitness will be influenced to some degree by prevailing social trends (compare, for instance, pictures of Western women in the Victorian era, the 1960s and the 2000s). The very idea of fitness cannot be entirely separated from fashions in body shape, the sorts of physique needed to enable a person to take part in popular pursuits, and trends in preventive medicine and health education. Thus, a statement 'Andy has optimum physical fitness' will rest both on statistical comparison and human definition and social trend.

2 *Advice to exercise can lead to undesirable consequences.* Not everybody wants to exercise. Some people find the activity boring, tiring, painful or just a waste of time. It is not inconceivable that constant advice to exercise might force people into doing something, perhaps trying jogging, against their real wishes. What's more, if people consistently refuse to exercise despite well-meaning pressure, advice to exercise could create guilt, stress and unnecessary anxiety about the damage not exercising could be doing. Moreover, there are significant risks of addiction, injury and even death – associated with exercise.[66] Advice to exercise does not lead to desirable ends in every case.

An illustration of the extent to which values permeate health work interventions: the health visitor, the doting daughter and the *Sporting Life*

Carole, a health visitor in the Handsworth area of Birmingham, UK, cares for an elderly woman called Veronica, who lives with her daughter Maggie. Carole has worked in the area for just over 3 months. She is 25 and, despite her demanding job, still rather shy and reserved. Carole's parents have lived in Harborne (a prosperous area of Birmingham, markedly different

An illustration of the extent to which values permeate health work interventions: the health visitor, the doting daughter and the *Sporting Life* (Continued)

from Handsworth) for 23 years, and Carole has not yet left home. She reads the *Daily Mail*, always dresses 'smartly and sensibly', and could be classified as 'lower middle class' (both her parents are school teachers). She hopes soon to move from Handsworth to a more rural 'patch'.

Veronica and Maggie live in a Victorian terraced house which has been divided into two flats by their landlord. They have a feud with the couple who occupy the other flat, who (they say) do not keep their three Alsatian dogs quiet enough. Veronica's condition prompted the visit in question, since she had recently had a urinary infection, and her doctor thought it appropriate to keep a friendly eye on her progress.

Veronica is in her mid-seventies and, when Carole arrived, was sitting quietly in her armchair, slim with grey hair tied back in a neat pony-tail, with a grace and elegance that sometimes accompanies age borne stoically (*). Maggie the daughter, in blatant contrast, is short (less than 5 feet tall) and very fat indeed, almost comically round (*), behind huge owl spectacles. She is in her early thirties.

Carole spoke to Veronica, who tried to reply but was repeatedly interrupted by the ebullient Maggie. It was established – eventually – that the urinary infection and sporadic incontinence had greatly improved, and was no longer a worry. Instead, Maggie seemed obsessed with the desire to have her mother fitted with a hearing aid. Maggie's argument was that her mother had difficulty hearing some television programmes, although Carole could see she obviously had no trouble catching what her daughter was saying. Much to Maggie's irritation, Veronica steadfastly refused to try a hearing aid. She said she didn't want to be a nuisance, and anyway she didn't need one. Carole noticed, with regret, that Maggie treated Veronica as if she were a little girl, despite her still impressive manner and appearance (*).

Maggie was unstoppable on the topic of herself and her mother. She explained to Carole, who knew already, that both she and Veronica were dependent on the State for their income (*), and then introduced the six cats, each of which was contemptuously self-satisfied and very well fed (*). Maggie bubbled with news of her mother's recent medical history, and of her own career 'under the doctor' too. She was pleased – even proud – that she was to pay a visit to the surgery that evening. It seemed to Carole that her main motivation was her mother (*), which was rather a shame because Maggie was undeniably articulate and intelligent.

The consultation took place in an unashamedly grimy living room, which had not been cleaned or vacuumed for months. It smelt old-house musty, with a mingling of stale sweat and food. The room was untidy in every imaginable respect and, although only small for a living room, was home to an enormous electric fire, flanked by two equally intimidating television sets.

It was 3 o'clock in the afternoon. Carole had obviously interrupted Maggie during a meal since she could see, sitting at a dangerous angle atop a cluttered sideboard, a plate stacked high with chips, sausage, baked beans, lamb chops and gravy. Carole could not help thinking that 'a heart attack on a plate' was really the last thing Maggie needed in her obese state (*). And, in Carole's eyes, what was worse was that most of the papers littering the room were recent copies of the *Sporting Life* (*), a paper for horse racing punters. The latest edition lay open on the arm of a big soft chair – obviously Maggie's – placed only 3 feet away from the right-hand television (*). Maggie had been standing for the last few minutes, in which time two of the cats had moved in on the cushions, and another was eyeing the portable trolley by the side of the chair.

Carole looked for an opportunity to leave. She thought she might hasten her departure by offering to take Veronica's pulse. Maggie accepted this proposal on her mother's behalf – on

(Continued)

> **An illustration of the extent to which values permeate health work interventions: the health visitor, the doting daughter and the *Sporting Life* (Continued)**
>
> condition that she had her pulse taken as well – at which Carole was mightily relieved that she could at last do something vaguely medical. At least now she could say she had visited the family to further their health, or so she reasoned.
>
> As she left, Carole thought she would be very depressed if she had to live a life like that in conditions like those. At the very least she would have made the effort to de-clutter the place and redecorate in pastel shades (*).

Comment

The above situation is saturated with values and value judgements, some of the most obvious of which are indicated like this (*), but of course there are many others too. There is valuing of relationships (Maggie and Veronica), valuing of aesthetics (the appearance of Veronica, the appearance of the room), valuing of lifestyle (the horse racing hobby), valuing of cleanliness (or not), valuing of personal lifestyle, valuing of health (Carole's understanding of health is different from Maggie's – Carole would *never* eat like that for fear of the morbidities associated with obesity) and valuing of technique (the medical intervention as the pulse was taken). On top of these values there are specific moral judgements – judgements of right and wrong about which the three characters disagree. For instance, Carole is of the opinion that Maggie is morally wrong to treat her mother as she does (Carole also believes Maggie is morally wrong to treat herself as she does), while Maggie has no doubt that she is justified in her actions. And not only are statements such as 'Maggie is a bad daughter' value-laden, but far less overtly judgemental statements such as 'Maggie is overweight', 'Maggie eats unwholesome food' and 'Maggie's house is a mess' also have subjective content.

In the example, many of the value judgements will be reasonably clear to outside observers, though not so apparent to those directly involved. Value judgements such as these do not occur only in the context of professional health work interventions, nor only between people who come from different class backgrounds. On the contrary, value judgements are made in the great majority of human encounters, even those where people share the same values.

It is vital that health workers become more accomplished at recognising the varieties of values that come into play. Much bad feeling, and many disputes over 'moral matters', come about simply because alternative values are not recognised as potentially plausible possibilities (though seen through the eyes of someone who conceives of the world differently). Each side tends to regard their own position and outlook as right, and that of the 'opposition' wrong. Yet if the values are spelled out and clarified it becomes far easier to see the situation from other perspectives. (Is Carole totally correct in her view? Is Maggie truly mistaken – isn't she happy? Is she really morally wrong to act as she does? What are her priorities? Are they so unreasonable?) This way it becomes easier to gain a fuller picture of what is going on. It becomes possible to take a different way of thinking seriously and to appreciate why another person values something you do not – see **Chapter Eleven** in particular.

Evangelicism – a false start

Certain people are moral evangelists who attempt to find their way through the proliferation of values in two inadequate ways: by resort to rhetoric rather than reason, and by appeal to a single value, or set of values, as absolutely morally correct. Throughout the ages the moral evangelist's slogan has been 'there is no alternative'.

An example

In 1986 there was (in Britain) a well-publicised controversy over the rights of parents to be informed, by general practitioners, if an under-age daughter requests contraception (the legal age for consent to sexual intercourse in the UK is 16). The issue hinged on the question of whether or not parental consent is necessary. Mrs Victoria Gillick, a self-appointed campaigner for parents' rights, wanted to protect the authority of parents over their offspring. Her position – which she said was the only morally tenable one – was that sexual intercourse under the age of consent is unequivocally wrong. From this she went on to insist that anything that encourages it (for instance, the prescription of contraceptives) must be bad, regardless of any other good that might come about (a reduction in teenage pregnancy, for example).

Mrs Gillick gave us a classic example of moral evangelism. However, ethical extremists do not belong exclusively to right-wing political groups or religious persuasions. There are, for example, many left-wingers who are just as dogged. The Labour MP Clare Short once famously introduced a bill to outlaw the publication of pictures of topless women in newspapers. She argued that such pictures exploit women and encourage male violence. Her argument has merits, in my opinion, but it is not the only morally supportable view, and there is evidence both for and against it.

Moral evangelists picture controversies as stunningly clear-cut. For them, there is always one entirely correct position (their own) while every other option is equally wrong. The moral evangelist understands morality only in the dramatic sense. It is her misfortune to be able to see only the tip of the iceberg. Indeed, the evangelist misses so much it is tempting to conclude that she hardly discerns the moral issues at all.

Can value conflicts be resolved in a more satisfactory way?

There are five conceivable routes towards the resolution of value conflict – five paths to consider in the search for the truly moral:

1 Finding some ultimate value or ultimate ordering of values – the quest for objective morality

It is commonly believed that some acts are so obviously ethically correct that any sane person must define them as moral. For example:

- The absolute truth should be told at all times.
- Professionals are morally obliged to perform their duties to the best of their ability.
- Never do anybody any harm in health care.
- At all times the health worker must encourage the maximum possible autonomy in the lives of everyone with whom she deals.

It is further imagined that several such 'ethically correct' statements can be combined to form an objective moral system.

Analysis

The four statements above are among the most frequently outlined moral principles in medicine and health care. However, by careful analysis, it is possible to show that they are questionable, and that their morally authoritative appearance is deceptive.

There are at least three ways to analyse statements of this sort.

Way one
The apparent maxims can be examined individually. To illustrate with the first: is it certain that a health worker should tell the truth in *all* cases? The answer is hardly clear-cut. Indeed, it is not always obvious what the truth *is*. Which writer on nutrition should the health worker refer to for his advice to the client? Which authority on immunisation should the health carer consult? How probable must a diagnosis be to be described as true? Is the truth about HIV and AIDS the same in 2008 as it was in 1988?[67]

It has been argued that there is a difference between 'telling the whole truth' and 'giving a client a true picture'. Much health work involves specialist knowledge, and Western medicine is based on the study of complicated scientific disciplines. To tell the client 'the whole truth' about a particular condition, to explain the biochemistry, the physiology and the histories of like conditions in other people, might not be feasible. There may be little time, and a proper understanding might require the client to have considerable prior knowledge. Inevitably, the most pertinent points have to be selected by the health worker. Furthermore, it may be her opinion that the client has been given a 'true picture', but her opinion will not necessarily be shared by a different health worker, even from a similar background.

A related complication concerns the extent to which a health worker should be honest about her true feelings. What if she thinks her patient is obnoxious and idle? To tell the whole truth in these circumstances would mean telling a client her opinion about him, and this is unlikely to be the best way to encourage his recovery.

Further uncertainty can occur if a health worker has factual information that might be detrimental to a client, or that he is holding in confidence. For instance, a health worker might be aware that a client's wife is seeing another man, and knows this is a significant factor in explaining the wife's recent offhand behaviour, which is depressing the husband and causing him to smoke more heavily than usual. In this case the information held by the health worker is both true and relevant to the client's health concern, but should it be conveyed? It seems impossible to argue that it is unambiguously right that it should.

Way two
The maxims can be applied to specific situations to see how they work out. Consider, for instance, the apparently moral statement: at all times the health worker must encourage the maximum possible autonomy in the lives of everyone with whom he deals.

It is not difficult to imagine real situations in which this expression is, at best, uncertain. Suppose you are introduced by a friend (who knows you are a health professional) to an acquaintance of his who has been taking a range of drugs, now wants to move on to heroin, but is uncertain of the safest way to inject himself. He has read about the drug and its risks and claims he has made an autonomous choice to experiment with it. As a health professional, do you encourage him in his decision (perhaps even injecting the heroin for him) or do you inform the police? If you justify a decision to tell the police by arguing that this will ultimately encourage the drug-taker's autonomy in the future (on the ground that if he is prevented from using drugs he will eventually have a wider range of opportunities from which to choose) you will still have acted against the statement in the short term (and a drugs conviction may close more doors than it opens). To give another example, how can the dictum be obeyed by a health worker who knows that a man has a sexually transmitted disease and is taking sexual partners without informing them of his condition? How is this man's freedom to direct his life to be encouraged without decreasing the autonomy of his unsuspecting partners?

Way three
A third method of analysis is *to study apparently objectively moral maxims in the light of other ethical theories.* Knowledge of these alternative theories should temper any tendency to make sweeping, unreflective statements. Given a decent understanding of technical ethics, any statement can be assessed from the point of view of any ethical theory, to see whether that particular theory would uphold or reject it. For example, a utilitarian health professional might well take issue with the position that the guiding principle of health work is to harm nobody. A utilitarian might believe that in many cases it is right to harm some people in order to ensure the maximum benefit for the remainder.

2 Finding a set of rules – the quest for a binding moral code

Some people think inquiry in ethics is nothing more than a matter of finding the proper set of moral rules. Their idea is that once the right rules have been uncovered there will be no unresolvable ethical problems. But this point of view is mistaken. Ethics cannot be adequately undertaken merely by following rules.

Throughout history most moral philosophers have held that ethics has a connection with rules and rule-following, but only a few have argued that the ultimate goal is to generate universally applicable rules. Certainly, much ethical inquiry is aimed at the justification of ways of acting that, if well-formulated and consistently followed, can guide civilised human conduct, but this is not the complete story. It is an error to expect moral philosophy to come up with a set of statements – some sort of Midas formula – that will always turn a tough dilemma into a golden solution. A more achievable aim of ethical exploration is the clarification of thinking, arguments and problems, the disclosure to decision-makers of the full range of possibilities open to them, and the elucidation of different points of view and ways of reasoning.

The flaw in thinking that ethics is only a question of finding the right rules is that there are no rules capable of providing the best answers to all possible life situations – no moral principles that can be sensibly applied across the spectrum of human experience.

No moral rule exists that cannot be justifiably broken

Take any example of an apparently binding moral rule, and it should not be too difficult to imagine circumstances in which it would be better to transgress it. It is, for instance, widely accepted that it can sometimes be better to lie than tell the truth, and robbing the rich to feed the poor has an established moral pedigree. Even working for health is not a binding rule since a person has to make a commitment to do this, and may decide it is not a path she wants to follow.

Never murder (where murder is defined as the intentional killing of another human being) looks, at first sight, to be a universal rule, but even this dictum can be legitimately ignored in certain circumstances. (Not everyone will agree that murder can be justified of course, but the point is that morally plausible defences of murder can be offered.) Capital punishment (the intentional killing of another human being, sanctioned by law) used to be morally acceptable in all European societies, but now is not. However, the majority of citizens, when polled, are in favour of it, and are therefore in favour of break-ing the moral rule 'never murder' in certain circumstances (a majority is usually found to be in favour of murder in wartime, in self-defence and in defence of property too).[68]

Euthanasia is said to be murder by those opposed to it (and by most legal systems in the developed world), yet is mercy-killing to its advocates. Whatever one labels it, eutha-nasia is intentional killing that some would allow and others prohibit – and this surely brings the moral status of the dictum 'never murder' into question.

Rules of games and rules in ethics are not synonymous

In competitive games, such as cricket and soccer, binding rules are essential. Without rules to give structure such games could not exist. The rules of cricket and soccer have been carefully developed in order to cater for every situation that might arise in a game. It is a prerequisite of playing such games that players agree that every rule is legitimate. Then, if they violate any, players must accept whatever punishment is laid down. In competitive games it is usual to have an independent judge whose role is to make sure the rules are followed.

Games are artificial, created by people who have defined the limits of each type of contest. A game is like a world apart. Within it, the rules are absolute and at least while the game is in progress there can be no outside interference with them.

Games are qualitatively different from ordinary life, which is not only vastly more com-plicated but not enclosed by unbreakable rules. Of course, human beings create moral rules just as we invent rules for games. However – unlike the rules of rugby or netball – moral rules are usually cast generally, and not spelt out to provide for all foreseeable situations.

Rules are a part of almost all daily behaviour, yet it is important to remember that there are many situations in which rules are not enough. Professional codes of practice are a good example. Codes of practice lay down general principles but cannot advise on their interpretation, explain how to decide between principles that conflict, or indicate when it is best to disregard them and deliberate independently. The following examples taken from codes of ethics show, without the need for any further comment, the extent to which their rules must be interpreted in context:

> Any act or advice which could weaken physical or mental resistance of a human being may be used only in his interest.[69]

> A doctor must always bear in mind the obligation of preserving human life.[69]

> Members will use appropriately their professional skills in the fulfilment of health education/ promotion activities which they believe to be effective.[70,71]

> A doctor must preserve secrecy on all he knows. There are five exceptions to this general principle:

> 1 The patient gives consent
> 2 When it is undesirable on medical grounds to seek a patient's consent, but is in the patient's own interest that confidentiality should be broken
> 3 The doctor's overriding duty to society
> 4 For the purposes of medical research, when approved by a local clinical research ethical committee, or in the case of the National Cancer Registry by the chairman of the BMA's Central Ethical Committee or his nominee
> 5 When the information is required by due legal process[69]

> Members will use their professional judgement regarding the confidentiality of information to which they have access, bearing in mind the requirements of the law and the best interests of their clients.[69]

It should be increasingly clear, as this search for morality develops, that health professionals not only need codes of practice (and a certain amount of legal knowledge) but also a decent acquaintance with ethical theory and modes of reasoning in general. Given this they can bow to or apply rules where they deem it appropriate, but are also able to apply well-reasoned personal judgement.

The trouble with rules can be summarised like this:

a. If the rules or codes are cast in general terms (for example, 'practitioners should always uphold the highest professional standards') they will either be open to wide interpretation or specific cases will contradict them: where exceptional action is needed morality can be increased by breaking the rules.
b. If the rules are specific it is inevitable that sooner or later cases will occur for which no rules have been laid down.
c. Even if *both* general and specific rules are decreed, problems (a) and (b) persist.

Rules should not be ignored in health work ethics

A continuum of positions on rule-following can be pictured. Dogmatically consistent rule-following at one extreme, arbitrary personal choice at the other. Neither of these poles is satisfactory if health work is to achieve the highest degree of morality.

To allow entirely free personal choice by health workers, not guided by rules, is not a workable policy. Health workers need the assurance rules can provide, and health services must operate with consistency if they are to secure public confidence. Furthermore, health workers are legally accountable for their actions, and most are understandably reluctant to do anything without the support of rules. Having said this, it is equally important that any code of practice or set of ethical principles should never be considered imperative.

Summary

The *benefits* of having rules and following them are:

a. If rules have been drawn up and agreed then it is likely they will be based upon considered reasoning and analysis
b. Rules provide useful guides for action
c. Rules will often be public – which means that those who are dealt with by health workers will know at least some of the rules.

The *disadvantages* of always conforming to rules are:

a. People's powers of judgement and decision-making tend to atrophy if not regularly used
b. Whatever the rules, situations will occur where breaking a rule will produce a higher degree of morality than abiding by it
c. A defining element of moral deliberation is that there must be uncertainty – at least at first. To state beforehand that a particular principle must be upheld whatever the circumstances is to negate morality. Without the possibility of choice moral deliberation is sterile.

3 Appealing to the law – the quest for moral legislation

Legality and morality – a tangled web

Legality and morality are not synonymous domains. Professional organisations recommend codes of practice to their members because many types of human conduct are potentially harmful, but do not break any law (being unreliable, being inconsistent, being vindictive, being friendly to some people and arrogant toward others, for instance). Such conduct is arguably unethical, but not illegal.

Lawful behaviours are frequently considered moral, and equally many illegal actions are deemed immoral. However, these are not the only possible classifications. There is a web surrounding this issue which, once untangled, can contribute toward a more complete understanding of what ethics is.

Clarification by separation

Note: laws vary between nations. Unless stated otherwise the laws referred to in this section are based on English law.

It is possible to make six basic distinctions. Acts may be judged to be:

a. Legal and moral
There are many examples in this category. For instance, most people agree that it is legal and moral to donate money to charity, to work voluntarily with disabled people, or to listen to another person as he relates his troubles. Indeed some moral actions are legally enforceable, though it is debateable whether actions done under duress can be said to be moral. For example, courts of law compel witnesses to tell the truth as they know it, and most contracts are legally enforceable, which is an official way to ensure people keep promises.

b. Legal and immoral
Morality can conflict with law. The following examples are arguably immoral, yet all are legal. It is necessary to concede the validity of one only in order to recognise the sharpness of the legal/moral distinction.

  i. When a person breaks a marriage vow
  ii. When a person makes a promise without intending to keep it
  iii. When a lecturer offers higher grades to a student than his work merits in return for sex
  iv. When government ministers cut the money available to higher education, and consequently deprive some people of education from which they could otherwise have benefited
  v. When a soldier kills a person in war
  vi. When a person is imprisoned purely as punishment, without attempt at education and rehabilitation
  vii. When governments deprive people of rights enjoyed by others
  viii. When people, acting under the law, intentionally physically or mentally disable other people. For example, it remains legal in some Arab states to cut off one or both hands of a person found guilty of stealing, and the possession of heroin carries a mandatory death sentence on conviction under Malaysian law.

c. Illegal and immoral
There are many examples of this combination, though in each case it is conceivable that some people will not agree that the acts are immoral. However, it can plausibly be said that burglary, intimidation, violence and reckless driving are both illegal and immoral.

d. Illegal and moral
Like the legal and immoral combination, this category can provoke debate, but it is not unreasonable to suggest that the following actions are both moral and illegal:

  i. When a driver breaks a speed limit in order to take a man suffering from a heart attack to hospital

ii. When a group obstructs city traffic by a 'sit-down' demonstration against the use of nuclear weapons

iii. When a person embezzles money from a wealthy company in order to donate it to children's charities

iv. When a charitable organisation breaks a country's import regulations in order to get life-saving food to starving people as quickly as possible

v. When a person employed by a welfare department interviews a claimant in obvious need, is prevented by a technicality from providing help, and yet falsifies certain of the claimant's details in order that the need can be met

vi. When a general practitioner fills out a sickness certificate falsely in order to help her patient. The doctor might, for instance, be unable to find any specific complaint but be of the view that the patient would benefit from time away from work pressures, and so reports a very general condition – stress, depression, or viral illness perhaps.

e. Legal and amoral

With this classification everything depends on the sense of morality invoked. If morality is conceived only in the dramatic sense (ethics at the tip of the iceberg) then most activities will be legal and amoral just because so many of them will not be thought to be in the ethical realm. However, if ethics is interpreted in the general sense – in which all activity has moral import – then few actions can be so described (see the **Preface to the Second Edition** for expansion of this point).

f. Illegal and amoral

As with the 'legal and amoral' classification everything depends upon the sense of morality in play. For example, if one takes the view that both intentions and consequences must be taken into account, an illegal act done in ignorance can be neither moral nor immoral. For instance, a tourist might park his car illegally in a foreign city without meaning to break any law or even realising he has done anything untoward, and without causing any other person harm. Or a person might genuinely forget to have her car checked for roadworthiness (a legal requirement in many countries) thus breaking the law, but not offending any moral standard (unless the view is taken that law sets the moral standard).

Figure 28 illustrates the six categories.

It ought now be easy to see that the quest to find the truly moral through legislation is doomed to failure. What is legal and what is moral are not necessarily related. It may be that a system of law is necessary to ensure minimal levels of morality and to maintain social order. But this is not to say that systems of law are therefore always moral systems.

4 Settling for relativism – giving up the quest

So far it has been shown that it is not possible to discover a single value that can be said to be objectively moral. Nor is it possible to invent rules or laws guaranteed to produce the most moral outcomes. And thus it might appear that the only solution is to succumb to relativism. But this is an inadequate answer too.

In order to explain relativism it is helpful to contrast it with objectivism.

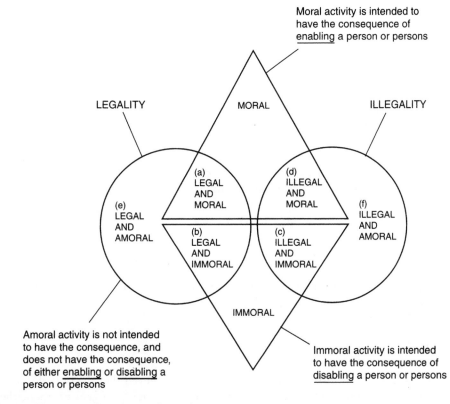

Figure 28 Distinguishing law and morality

Objectivism

There is a metre rule in Paris that sets the standard for any metre length. Objectivists argue that in most walks of life there are standards of truth analogous to the metre rule, even if it is not yet certain what they are. In science, for example, objectivists maintain that researchers are discovering truth about reality, truth about the world as it is independent of human interpretation. In the same vein, objectivists think different sorts of human society can be judged more or less primitive according to how rational they are. This view rests on an assumption that there is an objective standard of rationality to which some of the human race conform, and all should aspire to. Where societies are found to behave illogically or unreasonably when judged by the standards of anthropologists, objectivists claim these societies are irrational.

Relativism

Against objectivism, relativists insist there are no objective standards of truth. As far as human society is concerned relativists argue that different social systems operate according to non-universal standards, even though some standards may be held in common. One implication of this is that it is not only morally wrong but conceptually impossible to criticise them on the ground of irrationality. Since some societies operate with different forms of rationality, logic and truth, the anthropologist who assumes to judge an alien culture as 'irrational' or 'illogical' is able to do so only from the standpoint of his own cultural norms, not in line with an objective standard. For the relativist, if society does not conform to the norms the anthropologist calls rational then the other society is irrational only in the opinion of the anthropologist. Societies can be said to be irrational when compared to other societies, but this does not mean that the strange society is truly irrational because there is no external standard by which to judge this. Standards of truth are relative to different contexts.

These opposed positions conflict in moral philosophy too, as the following examples show.

Types of moral relativism

The following theories are relativist. None refers to an ultimate standard of morality, and each gains strength by denying its existence.

Emotivism

This point of view was put forward by A.J. Ayer,[72] who believed that the only difference between a statement describing facts and a statement offering a judgement about their morality is the personal opinion of the speaker. For Ayer the statement 'the nurse did not explain the likely side-effect of the treatment' can be distinguished from the statement 'the nurse was wrong not to explain the likely side-effect of the treatment' merely on the ground that the second statement has words added which express disapproval of the nurse's behaviour. This is a value judgement and, according to Ayer, it is not possible for people to contradict each other about statements of value because such statements have nothing to do with truth or falsity. Since everything in the realm of value is a matter of opinion, all one can do is continue to express one's opinions, and continue to give vent to one's emotions.

Furthermore, any apparently meaningful argument about an ethical issue can never be genuine since ethical judgements are kinds of feelings only, based ultimately on the psychological state of each interested individual. All that can be said of each feeling, each emotion and each value is that each is of exactly equal merit – all opinions are as good or as bad as each other, and since no moral standard exists outside emotion and feeling there is no yardstick against which to measure the differences. Which means, of course, that it is impossible to decide who is right in ethical disputes.

Where is this theory weak?
The trouble with this theory, as with all types of relativism, is that it fails to provide solid ground on which to stand. Not only does it deny the possibility of making moral judgements that can be said conclusively to be better than alternatives, but it implies that to respond according to one's feelings is as desirable as to respond using reason.

Although it is true that value judgements cannot be said to be true or false in the way a statement about the physical world can (just as it is not possible to say decisively that a particular painting or record album is aesthetically good or bad), it is insufficient to say that ethical disputes relate only to people's psychological states. While subjective opinion is an essential part of moral reflection, the real world and the outcomes of decisions taken in it are an integral part of ethics. To understand ethics properly is to recognise that there is more *at stake* than opinion and emotion: although it is not always possible to reach agreement about values it is often possible to discover which outcomes will most favourably affect those involved, and it is also possible to agree to try to find a workable consensus.

Egotism

Egotism is more an assertion than a theory, since it equates 'being moral' with the consistent pursuit of self-interest. The moral egotist asserts that what is morally good is what is in his interest: good is what is good for him. Achieving other people's interests is not an equivalent moral good.

Egotism has always been a mainstay of economic theory. The economist's 'rational man' is the self-interested man, the man for whom altruism and respect for others has little or no meaning. The 'rational man' takes other people into account only in so far as they are a threat and in competition for the scarce resources he covets. If morality has any meaning at all for this form of economics it exists only in relation to the desires of individuals.

Where is this theory weak?
One of the difficulties with arguing against relativism is that since he denies the existence of objective standards the relativist has only to state that his version is as good as any alternative. And as far as he is concerned he need not argue further. However, the relativist's opponent should not accept this tactic, but must insist on an examination of the theory's implications, and demand the fullest justifications for its premises. For instance, egotism must depend in some way upon psychology and genetics, which are open to debate and empirical test.

Most health workers will find the egotist account of morality alien since it is diametrically opposed to the values implicit in caring for others. Egotism denies that moral activity is a process of reflection and deliberation which must take account of other people as well as oneself, and as such it is difficult to see how it is a moral theory at all.

Cultural relativism

For the cultural relativist the question of what is morally right and wrong does not rest finally on the opinions or feelings of individuals. Instead, she believes that moral notions are generated by social arrangements, and that there is no yardstick beyond cultural standards. The ethical codes upheld in one society are not necessarily morally right in another, and it is impossible to decide which view is best. It has, for example, been documented[72] that Eskimos believed it to be morally correct for children to kill their parents while they were still able-bodied, to prevent them becoming senile and decrepit. For most Westerners such behaviour seems clearly immoral: the idea of children putting their parents to death is abhorrent (especially to parents), and remains abhorrent even when the justification for the behaviour is understood. It was apparently an Eskimo belief that people retain the physical bodies possessed at their death in the after-life. Consequently it makes sense to kill people (with or without their consent) in order to ensure they are not disabled in the next world. And that is where we must leave matters according to the cultural relativist. Since there is no such thing as objective morality there is no point in trying to arbitrate between the Eskimo and the Westerner.

It is taken for granted by many European citizens that the principles under which we have lived for generations are objectively good. Democracy, free speech, freedom from fear of death at the hand of another, freedom to own property and equality under the law are all popularly considered to be fundamentally moral principles. But the cultural relativist begs to differ. She points out that Europeans have not always held such values and may not hold them in the future. Furthermore, there are always some people who would change them because *they* do not regard them as the most moral possible. European morality is objective only in the sense that the majority of the people silently assent to it.

To different degrees, all types of relativism make the claim that the search for morality – at least for an external objective morality – is misguided. Paradoxically relativist theories can inspire the search for universal standards since they tend to inspire the inquirer to give reasons why a practice is morally better than another. Unless this is possible, unless some answer can be found to relativist scepticism, there is no difference between the statement 'you must not kill me because it would be immoral' and the statement 'you must not kill me because I don't want you to'. But there should be the world of difference between them. The first implies that to kill a human being is wrong because it offends against an important moral standard, while the second asserts that it is wrong to kill a human being only because he is interested in self-preservation.

We have an indefinite range of interests that are frequently in conflict. "What is needed is some set of standards to provide some arbitration – some sort of moral guidance – in cases where interests are in competition. Fortunately, there is a plausible answer to the relativist. It lies in an appeal to the facts."

*Note: I no longer think this statement is correct. It implies that the way to deal with moral relativism is to discover 'some set of standards' and/or 'facts' – but of course the relativist argument is correct. There simply are no such moral standards 'out there' to find. I now think we need: (a) transparent, reflective processes (**Chapter Eleven**) and (b) open commitment to theories of purpose – i.e. open explanations of why each of us believes in a particular way of living and acting (see the **Introduction to the Second Edition**).*

5 An appeal to the facts – the focus on what is

Before a path towards a more solid morality is mapped out it is necessary to introduce an important distinction, the distinction between what is and what ought to be the case.

The distinction between ought and is

"This distinction is introduced as a preliminary stage in an argument to pin down the source of morality (at least in respect to health work). The distinction shows that the very idea of morality is partly created by human beings. However, this does not imply that morality has no independent basis."

Note: This is wrong.

As we have seen, statements about morality are qualitatively different from statements of fact in that they can never be proven. Armed with this knowledge, it is possible to avoid the trap of thinking that evidence of what is is evidence of what ought to be.

Consider the following statements:

- Eric took $10 from his grandfather's wallet.
- Ian took the gun and shot John three times between the eyes.
- David donated $50 to Save the Children.
- Anne told a lie in order to spare her boyfriend's feelings.

Although it looks as if each statement has intrinsic moral substance, the is/ought distinction shows that the moral content is added by human beings. Without our opinions, impressions and judgements, each statement is nothing more than a factual report (so long as each statement is true). If we assume Eric was stealing, we might think he was morally wrong to take $10 from his grandfather's wallet. But nowhere in the act itself, or in the statement reporting the act, is it possible to discover rightness or wrongness, an 'ought' or an 'ought not'. The bare fact is that Eric removed money from a wallet. He might have been fetching it for his grandfather or borrowing it with permission, and even if he was stealing it the notion that 'stealing is bad' is a social judgement, not a natural fact.

What is just is, and it is not possible to argue validly from factual premises to moral conclusions. Whenever this is attempted the moral element is smuggled in like this:

Ian took the gun and shot John three times between the eyes.
Killing people is morally wrong.
Therefore Ian was wrong to shoot John three times between the eyes.
The first premise is factual, the second (in italics) is not.

How does this help inquiry into the ethics of health?

It is important in the following ways. First, it reinforces the point that there is no objective morality to be discovered in the sense that Mount Everest exists to be discovered. We cannot embark on experimental field trips to find out what is truly right – rather we must use reason. Second, the is/ought distinction can make us wary of arguing that because the group of human beings of which *we* are a part acts in a certain way (because the group is as it is) this is the most moral way to behave. Third, and most important of all, we can now begin to understand that although moral judgement has an essentially subjective component, this does not mean it is impossible to base moral principles on objective evidence. Although it is logically incorrect to derive an 'ought' from an 'is', it is not invalid to found a moral theory on matters of fact.

Let us see how this can be so. The moral quality of actions depends at least in part upon the value of what they bring about. In order to know whether some action is morally good it is therefore necessary to understand what is worthwhile in two factual senses:

i. It is necessary to understand what the people you will affect with your actions value (their values are subjective but *that* they value as they do is a fact).
ii. It is necessary to understand that people do not have infinite potential, though they can develop in a wide range of ways. Some of these ways (continuing to breath, not being in excruciating pain, being able to think) are absolutely necessary if they are to develop at all further. And some other ways (not being injured, not being seriously ill, not being ignorant) are necessary if their further development is to be fulfilling.

Moral actions must intend to promote what is good in one or both of these senses, though how to do this specifically for the best must be the subject of careful deliberation in each case.

Note: I still hold the above view, but it does not move the search for morality on very far. All it really says is that people are people, and if you value people then you must value their futures, in a very general way.

"Work for health is a fundamentally moral endeavour because it encourages both biological and chosen human potential."

Note: I no longer think that work for health is fundamentally moral, meaning that by doing work for health you are therefore objectively being moral. Yes, health work must in some way be to do with liberating potential – but there can be disagreements about the relative importance of human potentials, and what one person might regard as a healthy potential another might just as well regard as unhealthy.

This insight undermines the is/ought objection. Being human and possessing a range of worthwhile potentials is a fact which contains an ought. That is, the statement 'Fred is a human being' contains within itself the statement 'Fred ought to be a human being'. This cannot be denied without absurdity.

The precise moral importance of being human is less clear. This book contends that work for health makes the reasons it is valuable to be human explicit, and that those who decide to work for health make a basic moral commitment – uniting the ideas of health and morality.

This argument cannot be made quickly or easily, and has now been developed over several works; however, further support must be provided now. If it is true that morality cannot be discovered as Mount Everest can, and if it is true that there is no morality beyond human value and thought, morality must lie in what is of central importance to human beings, what human beings have in common – what human beings are for.

Note: Again, this is true in general, but the idea collapses as soon as specific human goals are stated – as everyone knows, people frequently disagree fundamentally about what human beings are for.

A search for immorality

Discovering the nature of morality by focusing on its opposite: immorality

Because there is a baffling variety of candidates for the title 'truly moral' and no uncontroversial criteria for judging between them, it is sensible to attempt to identify *immoral* actions in order to cast new light on their apparently polar opposite – the moral.

An example from social work

This strategy is common in social work, where there is often divergence of opinion about what constitutes a 'good parent'. Does a good parent leave his child in the care of others for long periods? Is the person who has little feeling for her child yet still provides diligently for all material necessities a good parent? Or does a good parent love her child so deeply that she will never let him out of her sight? It is hard to say which parent comes closest to 'the ideally good parent' because this label is so obviously contestable. However, what is important so far as this inquiry is concerned is that although there is endless controversy about the definition of 'good parent', it seems possible to reach universal (or almost universal) agreement about what a bad parent is. For example, it would be very difficult to find a social worker who does not agree that a person who consistently and deliberately inflicts physical and mental harm upon her child, who never considers what might be good for him, and does not intend to produce long-term good either, is a bad parent.

On the objectively immoral: Grand Thiam

"The following hypothetical society is described for two reasons: to give a clear example of immorality and to draw attention to an association between the ideas of health and liberty. If this illustration is thought too fanciful it will be rendered relevant by relating it to real families, familiar relationships, politics and behaviours in the workplace, or to societies unable or unwilling to provide fulfilling work for many of their people."

   Note: The argument in the Third Edition is that there are no 100% clear examples of immorality.

The way of things in Grand Thiam

Grand Thiam is a human civilisation that has either existed in the past or will exist in the future – it does not matter which. Despite enviable material wealth its residents are becoming vociferous: demanding power, demanding greater liberty and demanding the right to decide their own destinies.

This pressure for change is a serious threat to the government's priorities. Grand Thiam is ruled by 100 Elders not allowed to marry or procreate, but who can select their successors without public consultation. For them the ideal society has strong social cohesion, every citizen knows his place in it, there is unquestioning obedience to the law, all industry is able to achieve maximum productivity and disease is kept to a minimum. They prefer these values over such alternatives as free and uncensored speech, public participation in decision-making and equal opportunity of access to political power. From the Elders' point of view, the more such values proliferate the more the *status quo* is threatened.

Through a recently developed cocktail of genetic and educational manipulation the Elders now have the power to engineer their perfect world.

Dwarfing

Time has moved on and the Elders have used the technology. The 'educational' part of the process made use of a Platonic 'noble lie'. All history books were destroyed and replaced by texts that indoctrinated the belief that a caste system is the only possible pattern on which an orderly society can be based. This propaganda was reinforced by genetic engineering – the insertion of the donkey's 'subservience' gene into human embryos – and the addition of chemicals to the water supply, intended to alter mental states and attitudes. In the early years the plan was effected by weakening the population's curiosity, logical power and questioning abilities through 'immunisations' universally administered, and by radically increasing the banality of television programmes and newspapers. As the population who had experienced relatively unfettered thought died off the manipulations were stepped up, so all new citizens could be physically and intellectually fitted from birth for their allotted roles (which were defined by various sub-committees of a working party of the Elders' steering group). This not only meant that people's intellectual powers were reduced and clouded, but also that the physiques of some were artificially restricted. The Elders' aim was to ensure the creation and perpetuation of their 'ideal state' through restraining the very existences of the human beings who constitute it.

It was necessary to interfere with the physical development of some children in order to suit them physically for the tasks they were to take on in 'adult' life. This meant that for some jobs, such as the non-automated inspection of pipelines, the cleaning of tower blocks and skyscrapers, and some types of mining, the physical development of some children was halted before puberty, and their intellectual development regulated according to the complexity of the task they were to perform. (If this seems incredible it is salutary to remember the not uncommon practice in India for desperate parents to cripple and mutilate their offspring in order to enable them to beg more successfully.) Many of Grand Thiam's children were intentionally prevented from fulfilling their natural physical and mental potentials in the interest of the society as a whole, as this interest was perceived by the Elders. In other words, these children were deliberately dwarfed.

A major connection: health work is work against dwarfing

"There is something intuitively disgraceful about the process of dwarfing."
   Note: Unfortunately, this does not seem to be everyone's intuition.
   Analysis of the theory and practice of health work shows that its underlying sense is the concern to remove or prevent obstacles to physical and mental growth. Health work strives to enable people to bring to fruition the range of potentials that lie latent within them. By educating, by curing disease, by mending broken bones, by developing personal power to conceive – to picture one's situation and future possibilities more clearly – health work is the antithesis of dwarfing.
   "Since it is an exact counterbalance to dwarfing (or 'the immoral') it follows that the health work endeavour is as objectively moral as it is possible to be. But because there are different types of health work, different senses of moral, and an indefinite range of contexts and ways in which health work can be carried out, it is not possible to say definitely that a particular intervention is *ideally* moral. It is also a mistake to assume that each attempt to create health will be as moral as any other. As was shown in the two situations involving the young footballer with a broken wrist (now précised in the **Introduction to the Third Edition**) there are degrees to which the enabling (or anti-dwarfing) can be carried out. However, if the intent of the health worker is to enable the enhancing potentials of the person she is working with, if the path she pursues is one which she can justify with integrity, then the work will inevitably be moral."
   Note: I continue to believe that there is something vitally morally important about working for health, and I would advocate to anyone that they adopt a foundationally health promoting approach to life. I just cannot prove this to someone who takes a different view – I can argue for it extensively, but if she does not share my beliefs I will never convince her.
   In the ailing paradigm there is a massive imbalance between the attention given to the physical and all other aspects of people's lives – even though it should be quite clear that the subject matter of genuine work for health is not just bodies but whole people and the external factors that make up their lives. Work for health should be the comprehensive construction and maintenance of the foundations on which people can achieve. In the new paradigm no *bona fide* health worker will seriously take the view that the end point of health work is nothing more than a non-diseased body. It will be a commonplace that health work does not strive to keep people alive as an end in itself – it does not work only on bodies and treat people as objects. Instead, it will be recognised that a body is given therapy in order to allow the person to go on making real as much of his fulfilling potential as possible.
   Work for health can properly be so much more than medical and hospital care and traditional health education – yet the old paradigm is stubborn and hard to shift. It is easy enough to explain this inertia, but very much harder to do anything about it. For example, it is presently uncontroversial that children's eyes should be checked at an early age. The only debate is about how early this should be. Many health authorities recommend that children should have had their eyes examined by the age of 3½, though some specialists argue that even this could be too late to remedy certain defects.
   Defects of vision can be detected and something practical can often be done with immediate effect. This is what the old paradigm is good at. Yet there is in principle no

reason why a person whose intellect has stagnated at 36 as a result of a tedious job and unchallenging existence should not be equally a target for a health intervention. A person's intellect is just as much a part of him as his eyes, and its flourishing is arguably even more important if he is to become a mature and interested person. The problem with health work is that the values, political judgement and empirical evidence involved with intervening with intellectual development are far more obvious, and the options more contentious, than with work with eyes and other physical features. But though this may be a *difficulty* it does not mean that such work is not genuinely part of the endeavour to create more health. In many medical consultations, in conversations between nurses and patients, in some types of health education, in women's health groups and neighbourhood schemes this endeavour is already going on. The extra needed to bring about the best version of the new paradigm is for the health service to acknowledge explicitly the breadth of health work, and to make clear the inescapable conclusion that work for health – within certain legal and moral limits – is work to liberate the fullest possible spectrum of human potential.

An objection

It might be argued that although the above account gives a credible view of health, it misunderstands the nature of potential. Because human bodies develop throughout life there are always biological potentials that can be enabled. But this is not so clear in the case of intellectual potentials. It might, for instance, be argued that schooling stops at 16 because only a minority of people have the potential for higher education, just as only a small minority of people can become athletes or cricketers.

Against this it can be said that the assumption that only physical potentials continue to develop throughout life is based on poor evidence. Work in psychology, psychiatry and education clearly shows the range of intellectual potentials that can be enabled throughout life. And there is considerable further evidence that development in logic and reasoning can be impeded (or dwarfed) through lack of practice, lack of expertise and lack of information.

In short, the problem is this: we have, in developed countries at least, no difficulty in accepting that a "working-class" child's broken leg should be set so that it will develop well, as it would have if it had not been injured. It is also self-evident that physical obstacles of this sort are not dealt with only for their own sake – only because they are injured, painful or abnormal. They are, of course, tackled in order to restore normal biological functioning, but are also dealt with so that a person can go on to live a fulfilled existence. People are not put back on their feet just for the sake of it, but in order that they can do more and be more satisfied. Physical potentials are enabled in order that further enhancing physical and mental potentials will be liberated as well.[8]

However, although the logic is identical, it is apparently more difficult to accept that: (a) the intellect of the child with the broken leg should be encouraged to develop as it would have given the educational opportunities at home and school that more privileged children have; (b) the child's emotional development should be brought to the level it could have been were it not for the disabling effect of his parents' broken marriage; or (c) the child's ability and opportunity to choose throughout life should be encouraged to flourish as fully as possible. But genuine work for health is work directed against the intentional or accidental dwarfing of people. And since every aspect of a person's being is potentially dwarfable, work for health should be correspondingly comprehensive.

Summary

A number of possible paths towards the discovery of the truly moral have been discussed and rejected in this chapter. What remains is the knowledge that it is necessary to consider human nature and potential empirically, in order to better understand what human beings are for, and so to learn how we should behave toward each other. Although it is impossible to give an objective list of enhancing potentials, and not possible to define what is truly moral, it is possible to be clear about what is immoral. This and the implicit notion of dwarfing are vital clues.

The following points have become clear:

1 There is no morality independent of human beings. What would such a morality be like? The claims of some religious groups that ethical rules have been established by a supernatural entity are opinion only and cannot be tested. If one believes that a deity creates morality then everything is evidence for this, yet if one chooses to disbelieve the claim then nothing counts as evidence for it. Crucially, since there is no evidence that would sway a neutral, the view cannot be empirically sustained. Surely the only possible place to search for morality is in the human race itself.

2 Any opinion of any human being about what is moral and what is not will always be challengeable. It is always possible to advance alternative opinions. This is part of the diversity of human thinking. And because there is such variance it is not enough even to search for common opinions shared by all human beings. It is impossible to discover values about which all human beings will agree. Not even seeking to avoid pain and treasuring one's own life can be said always to be universal human values. Athletes seek pain in order to push themselves towards higher performances, and people sometimes commit suicide. However, since these basic values will normally be shared, they do form part of the story about morality.

3 The fundamentals of morality lie in the fact of human existence, in what is naturally human. And it is at this point that the notion of health can be seen to be central to ethics. Human beings have certain physiological and mental potentials common to us all. If these are not allowed to develop in certain people then these people cannot be considered full persons. What is a human being for? The only way to answer this question is to give a list of potentials. Some of these, the very potentials on which health work should concentrate, are essential to being a person.

4 "Based on the three stages above, and the insight that the achievement of human potential is central to both health and morality in the richest sense (the sense that incorporates the complete iceberg – see the **Introduction to the Second Edition**), it is possible to develop an argument that the fullest degree of morality – or the most ethical intervention – is that which enables persons to achieve the fullest enhancing potentials of which they are capable."

Note: This argument breaks down because there will always be disagreement about the specific meaning of 'achieve the fullest enhancing potentials of which they are capable'. Simple as that.

Summary (Continued)

More substance yet needs to be added to this theoretical analysis. In order to be clearer about practical and moral priorities in work for health it is necessary to understand what people – or 'persons' in more technical language – actually are.

Conclusions

In earlier editions this chapter attempted to prove that work for health is a moral endeavour. It claimed that there is a fundamental connection between 'work for health' and 'creating morality'.

Speaking very generally, I still believe this. But while the idea may help some people understand just why work for health can be so morally inspiring, it does not help people make practical decisions where there is disagreement about the best way to resolve a situation.

To understand more fully the revised position of the Third Edition, readers should refer to the **Introduction to the Third Edition.**

Persons and Potentials

Introduction

We need a plausible working definition of 'person' to enable us to understand better the nature of those beings for whom health is so important, and to be clear what makes them special. Defining 'person' is a philosophical challenge with significant practical implications. For example, decisions about whether to switch off life support machines rest on a definition of personhood. They may not depend on this alone, but if a body has no prospect of regaining essential personal characteristics this is usually a decisive consideration.

John Harris's argument: towards a working definition of basic 'personhood'

Like philosophers before him, Harris[74] uses 'person' technically, out of line with ordinary use (where it means human beings after infancy). He argues that a person must possess features that make her existence valuable to her. It is not necessary to be human to possess these features (there may be persons on other planets who are not human) nor does it follow that a human being is automatically a person.

Harris quotes John Locke, who also wanted to distinguish persons from other creatures:

> We must consider what 'person' stands for; which, I think, is a thinking intelligent being, that has reason and reflection, and can consider itself, the same thinking thing, in different times and places; which it does only by that consciousness which is inseparable from thinking and seems to me essential to it; it being impossible for anyone to perceive that he does perceive.[75]

Locke's point is that although it is impossible for a person to 'perceive that he does perceive' in so far as seeing is concerned – one cannot see oneself seeing – a person can be aware of himself thinking (just as a person can be aware of his own rational fields – see the **Introduction to the Third Edition**). Locke recognised a condition now generally considered integral to personhood: self-consciousness – the awareness that enables an individual to 'consider itself, the same thinking thing, in different times and places'.

Harris thinks this a necessary condition too, but wishes to expand the concept. For Harris, if a human being is to be classed as a person it not only has to be self-conscious but must have the capacity to value its own life. Hence he unites two conditions: in order for a being to value its own life it has to be aware it has a life to value. This gives a simple definition – a person is 'any being capable of valuing its own existence'.[74]

'Persons' and 'full human beings'

Harris discusses an objection offered by Mary Warnock, who resists the use of 'person' on the grounds that it is confusing and could be used as a smokescreen to permit any action on any being so long as it does not count as a person. Warnock prefers the term 'full human being' instead. She thinks membership of the human species the vital moral principle, while Harris favours his version because it avoids 'speciesism' (discrimination between species).

Both 'person' and 'full human being' are meant to offer basic identifying criteria. But neither suggestion goes far enough. Neither stipulates a fulfilled human being – or a 'full person' – yet this is a vital step in the creation of a practical philosophy of health.

To be a full human being, or to have the capacity to value oneself, is only part of what is meant by being a full person

The principle of equal respect for persons is of central importance to health work and rests on the fact that some features of human existence are shared equally by us all. However, health work at its richest includes not only the obligation to treat people with equal respect and serve needs first where possible, but also to create and respect autonomy. Therefore it is necessary to construct a notion of 'full personhood', in order to include these additional concepts.

Harris's account of the value of life is made in a book about medical ethics – a tip of the iceberg text to do with hard life and death choices. His basic question is: what is it that makes life valuable at all? His answer refers to an elementary, abstract potential: people have the capacity to value their lives, and do so because they know their lives hold worthwhile future choices. According to Harris, to deny these possibilities to an individual who finds his life valuable is fundamentally wrong. And this is where the argument stops. Indeed this is as far as it is necessary to go for the purpose of helping clinicians and managers make moral decisions according to Harris's conception of morality. But – and this point bears repeating until it gains general acceptance – *the ethics of medical work is part of the ethics of health, but is not the whole story.* In order to contemplate the ethics of health properly it is necessary to consider what people's future choices might actually be. For Harris's purposes this is not important – all that matters is that there are some rather than no choices for the person. The ethics of health work, on the other hand, is interested in practical detail. The health worker must carefully consider – in theory and in context – the *nature* of the future choices she might enable.

Potentials

At this point it would perhaps be nice to be able to give a list of good and bad human potentials. But things are not this simple. People value different ends, our circumstances are enormously varied, and no two individuals are exactly alike – so a comprehensive list cannot be given. However, when considering persons in the context of health work in its richest sense, an important distinction can be made. It is possible – and necessary for the foundations theory of health – to distinguish between the notion of human potential in the abstract and in practice.

Human potential in the abstract

This idea inspires the Harris version of personhood. Even without reference to actual people it is possible to say that all persons – and those with the capacity to be persons – have potentials. Harris believes the capacity of a being to value its own existence is the most fundamental, but there are others too. For instance, all persons must have the capacity to think and reflect, and all living human beings' bodies must develop – all human beings have biological potential. It can also be said abstractly that some of these potentials will almost always be more desirable than others. For instance, ageing without physical pain is usually preferred to a life of agony. And it is normally thought better that a person values his life because he looks forward to future opportunities, rather than merely because his life exists.

Although it is infuriatingly difficult to specify which potentials should be considered good and which bad, the fact that all persons possess aspects of life in common makes a powerful claim possible. Although the precise degree to which interventions are moral can never be clear, it is nevertheless apparent that to prohibit the achievement of basic potentials in some people and not others is selective dwarfing, and as such can be considered immoral according to many ethical outlooks (but not objectively so – see the **Introduction to the Third Edition** and **Chapter Four**).

Specific human potentials

Good practical work for health depends upon the empirical investigation of actual potentials. Taking into account the two following conditions – that wherever possible the achievement of a desired potential in an individual should not decrease her future enhancing potentials, and that the achievement of the desired potential should not be at the expense of avoidable dwarfing in other people – it falls to the health worker (committed to the foundations theory of health) to consider with the client which of a range of possible potentials should be made reality. Sometimes the decision will be relatively simple. For instance, if a patient has broken his leg the prime consideration will be the restoration of its normal biological potentials. During treatment it may be possible to realise other potentials, dependent on the skill and vision of the health worker concerned. For example, the patient's confidence, knowledge and understanding might be increased by appropriate kindness, empathy and education.

In the care of terminally ill people the identification of achievable potentials is often less complicated because time is short and possibilities limited. Much depends on the choice of the patient, and hard decisions sometimes have to be made about the balance between the elimination of pain and the extent to which the patient is able to communicate with those he loves and who love him.

The most baffling choices face health workers who deal with people who have innumerable potentials, only some of which will ever become reality. If health workers are consistently to work in accord with the richest health work rationale they must take this range into account. Even if the complaint is a simple physical one, the best health worker will also seek to explore the client's feelings and future possibilities, viewing his life as a whole: does the client need help with a housing problem? Does he need advice about where to find friends? Will he benefit from an opportunity to take a programme of education? Does he have a sporting ambition or talent which is not being expressed? Does he have a creative ability or interest which might be developed by appropriate training and opportunity?

Only under an impoverished view of health work are these potentials not thought proper health work. To understand why more limited views of health are impoverished one need only ask: why is it important to cure disease – is it so that the morbidity statistics can be improved, or is it so that a person can go on to achieve in his life? How does it make sense to think that the physical aspects of human existence are the most important when the very features that mark off persons from other beings are our capacity for reason, for conceiving intellectually, for valuing our own lives, and for autonomous development?

Work for health is work to create full persons in a much deeper sense than Harris's elementary idea of personhood, and Warnock's notion of a full human being.

Dewey's idea of personal growth as the only true moral end

John Dewey was one of the few major philosophers to take a deep interest in education, which he considered a central *raison d'être* of philosophy. He believed that 'morals' is 'education', in the general senses of both words. Both notions, he thought, are inseparable from the idea of growth in a child. The end or purpose of the educational process is not something extra to this: 'Growth itself is the only moral end.'[76]

In Dewey's view people are best equipped to realise their individual capacities within a democratic society because:

> All social institutions have a meaning, a purpose. That purpose is to set free and develop *capacities* [my italics] of human individuals without respect to race, sex, class or economic status. And this is all one with saying that the test of their value is the extent to which they educate every individual into the full stature of his possibility. Democracy has many meanings, but if it has a moral meaning, it is found in resolving that the supreme test of all political institutions and industrial arrangements shall be the contribution they make to the all-round growth of every member of society.[76]

Dewey makes an important and comprehensive statement. His words are general and idealistic, but no less valuable for that. His sentiment is entirely in keeping with the spirit of this book. To paraphrase: Dewey's argument is that in a democracy any social institution (whether it is work, school or the family, for instance) is only moral in so far as it is directed towards the growth, in every possible way, of each unique individual in that institution, regardless of race, age, sex, class or economic status. Any social institution is valuable in proportion to the degree to which it helps every individual, equally, to achieve his or her fullest potential – to flourish – as comprehensively as possible.

Within certain limits[27] this noble aim is precisely what a foundational health service should aspire to. Any 'health service' that sets its sights lower than this – for whatever reasons – is not a health service in the most humane sense of the word. Any 'health service' that does not set out to encourage the development of full persons (Dewey's 'flourishing human beings') will exhibit some degree of morality, but not the fullest degree. It will not be the best possible health service, and will be part of a correspondingly less valuable society.

A difficulty

Once again the problem of discovering a set of values on which all can agree has appeared. It is probable that to those of a socialist or liberal persuasion Dewey's fine rhetoric sounds convincing. Yet it will seem nothing more than words without substance to a person whose views are influenced by the politics of the right.

The question of which potentials should be enabled is clearly a political issue. In a society motivated by individualism it might appear desirable to encourage the potential to be self-seeking. But in a society based on a more communitarian rationale it might not.

Different versions of health care can be arranged along a spectrum of types. At the one end health care might be devoted solely to the prevention and elimination of disease and illness, its only function to return bodies to a state where they can again be economically productive, or to make sure that illness does not restrict their abilities to produce. Between the poles health care might treat people as individuals in their own right, but only up to an imprecise and variable limit. And at the other end of the spectrum a health service might be based on the ideology that inspires Dewey, and might limit its resources only when the national budget has been exhausted.

Summary

'Person' is a technical term used by philosophers to describe beings with certain qualities, such as being self-conscious and valuing one's own life. However, in health work it can be enlightening to think of persons more broadly. For example, every person must have some potential for future development. Although the degree and type of future development varies enormously, in every person there exists the possibility to become more of what she could be. Foundational health workers should recognise the basic equality of persons, and should strive to ensure their maximum flourishing – paying the fullest attention to the talents and situation of all concerned.

Theories of Ethics

Introduction

This chapter offers an easy-to-read introduction to some well-established theories of ethics. Readers – especially students studying for practical health qualifications – are likely to find these explanations very helpful.

However, readers should be aware that in order to be a thoughtful, morally aware health worker, it is not necessary to know any ethical theory at all. It is much more important to understand yourself and your values, and to be prepared to learn and respect the values and decisions of others, as you gain experience.

Introduction to ethical theory

The essence of moral reasoning

Moral reasoning – the stamp of civilization – has been described as a prism able to shine a spectrum of light onto problems.[77] Which light gleams depends on who is doing the thinking. Moral reasoning requires knowledge, intelligence, patience and – from time to time – a will to compromise. Respect for it signifies personal maturity. It is not easy, but done properly moral reasoning is immeasurably better than bull-headed rule-following or mysterious intuition.

Thinking ethically

People who appreciate moral reasoning know rules and principles are both necessary and often conflict. Because of this, edicts and principles must be placed in context to see which are the most appropriate in a given situation. Such a judgement is easiest if the situation is analysed into key elements, the range of alternatives for action made apparent and their pros and cons assessed.

Any course chosen must be justified. This is traditionally done by appeal to principle or by emphasising the benefit of the expected outcome (or both). Furthermore, the committed moral reasoner does not make ad hoc decisions. She is concerned to choose in the light of previous decisions, and will also want to examine her present solutions with hindsight.

The Ethical Grid – an instrument designed to enhance moral reasoning – is introduced in **Chapter Nine** as a guide to health workers who would like to be ethically proficient. It incorporates the elements described above – and more – and is intended as a starting point for personal reflection and public debate. But first the ground must be prepared by reviewing classic theories of Western moral philosophy (some of which the Grid incorporates). The point of this – and of the Grid itself – is not to advocate a particular moral theory (which has been the dominant tradition in recent moral philosophy),[78] but rather to promote a general *way of thinking* amongst health workers.

A general distinction

The major division in Western moral philosophy is between deontology and consequentialism: between the opinion that morality depends on obedience to duties and the view that it rests on the calculation of costs and benefits. As the intricacies of moral philosophy unfold, this distinction can seem increasingly blurred. For example, some deontologists justify their stance on the ground that the consequences of abiding by principles are ultimately desirable, even if they do not maximise utility in the short term. And some consequentialists claim we are morally obliged to try to assess the consequences of our actions.

Deontology

(The word deontology is derived from the Greek word *deon*, and means study of duty.)

The central tenet of deontology is that a moral person must always do her duty. In its purest form deontology holds that a person should perform duties without exception, whatever the consequences. The nature of these duties is open to argument, since there is no principle on which all deontologists agree.

A deontologist might decide to adopt a single overriding duty – for instance, she might advocate that promises should never be broken, or that people should treat others as they wish to be treated themselves. Alternatively, the deontologist might adopt a range or hierarchy of duties to guide her actions. If so, in those cases where they conflict, she must decide which duties are most compelling. For example, a deontologist nurse might believe retributive justice (punishment for perceived wrongdoing) should be administered without exception, and that people should always keep promises. If she then promises a youth that whatever he tells her about what is depressing him will be kept confidential, and he tells her he has sold jewellery stolen from his mother, spending the money on fruit machines to feed his addiction to gambling, she has an impossible dilemma. On the one hand she is duty-bound not to break promises, yet on the other she believes wrongdoing should always be penalised. To decide which duties should take precedence in a case such as this, the deontologist has no choice but to engage in some form of moral reasoning, even if only to come up with a third duty to help her choose between the other two.

Deontological theories contrast with theories that take their guidance from the practical world (two examples are teleological ethics, which maintains that what ought to be done can be decided by studying what is good in fact, and utilitarian ethics, which holds that moral policies can be calculated by assessing happiness levels). Against these, deontological theories argue that the discovery of what is moral is never, or hardly ever, a matter for empirical research. On the contrary, the deontologist – dependent upon how pure a deontologist he is – will argue either that certain obligations and actions are right and good in themselves *regardless* of consequences, or he will say that although it is sensible to consider consequences some duties are nevertheless of supreme and abiding importance.

Most deontologists argue that it is wrong to ignore duties, even for temporary advantage. Ultimately, for deontologists, one should do one's duty because there are duties to be done – full stop.

Types of deontology

Act-deontology

Act-deontology is a rather puzzling version of deontology because it does not define its principles concretely. Indeed, act-deontology opposes rule-following, on principle. Sartre and other existentialists have been labelled act-deontologists because they place the focus of moral action not on rules or code books, but on human judgement in the context of each new situation. They assume that however much one situation might appear to resemble another each context and each actor is unique, and so each judgement about each solution should be unique too. A person judging now will be different, in so far as he will have had more experiences, than when he judged then. There are no standards other than the central conviction that everything in morality must rest upon the person who is to decide. Principles are not basic, although they can be considered. Consequences are not basic, although they can be taken into account. The decision-maker is basic. The single obligation of act-deontology is that a person should be true to herself.

Advantages of act-deontology

Act-deontology is not recommended for health workers enmeshed in the bureaucratic modern world. There must be overt rules and principles of conduct to guide professionals in complex organisations. However, act-deontology's emphasis on being true to oneself whenever moral deliberation is required should not be overlooked, even in the most codified organisations. Indeed, as we shall see, the spirit of act-deontology inspires the Ethical Grid.

Act-deontology draws attention to two important points. First, it reminds us that no moral rule can be applied with absolute confidence just because it has turned out well in the past. Each new situation – however similar it might appear to a past one – is unique (as time moves on people and circumstances change inexorably). Surprising things happen and hidden factors can come into play. Therefore it is morally inadequate to stick unthinkingly to rules and convention. Each circumstance is singularly alive and requires the fullest possible attention from the health worker. Simply to do what you have been told, or to carry out your work as if every single aspect of it is routine, is to shut your mind to the importance of yourself and the people in whose lives you intervene.

Second, act-deontology explodes the myth that a professional is somehow different from a non-professional. Pompous people think 'professional judgements' are different in kind from those made at home or on holiday. But act-deontology rightly insists that a person should be true to himself in every situation. Being a professional for a time is just another occasion in which authenticity is necessary. There are always choices to be faced: not least the choice between doing what one is contracted to do, and doing what one thinks ought to be done (a common tension for modern health professionals).

Disadvantages of act-deontology

Act-deontology is inordinately impractical. How can a system of care – or any other system for that matter – be built on a philosophy that advocates arbitrary decisions? While it is true that every situation in life must have distinctive aspects (even if only of time, place and participants) this is not the same as saying that *everything* about each situation will be unique. Indeed it can be deflating for a person – whether he realizes it as a child, an adolescent or in adult life – that there is nothing special about his life other than his own evaluation of it. The human condition is such that we are confronted with problems which are often horribly unique to ourselves, but it is rare for one person to experience a trouble that has not been suffered by many others. Because of this it is necessary to draw up rules – stronger than rules of thumb though not wholly fixed – to deal coherently with human problems.

Rule-deontology

Rather than insist that a person's moral choosing should depend on how she sees a situation at the time, the rule-deontologist asserts that moral decisions should be based on rules that should be followed whatever the likely outcome. Some rule-deontologists claim their rules are good in themselves while others – in a concession to consequentialism – claim the consequences of *not* acting according to them will be undesirable.

Advantages of rule-deontology

The chief advantage of rule-deontology is that the actions of those who espouse it will usually be predictable. Many codes of practice – themselves limited forms of deontology

– are in circulation in health services. The principles they contain are usually too general to ensure the predictability deontologists require. However, it would be possible for health service policy-makers to draw up more precise principles, which could be applied according to rule-deontology's intent. For instance, rules such as 'always tell the truth as you know it', 'always keep promises' and 'always respect other people as you would wish to be respected' could be fleshed out by means of detailed examples and case studies, and so become widely recognised principles of practice.

Disadvantages of rule-deontology

Rule-deontology's main problem is that if a single rule is chosen there will inevitably be occasions when it would be better if it were broken. And if a set of rules is chosen, then although the rules might appear to fit together in the abstract, sooner or later circumstances will reveal clashes between them. The trouble with rule-deontology is that it cannot offer guidance to the health worker who must choose between conflicting rules. Even if the rule-deontologist ranks the rules the first difficulty remains – there will be occasions when it will be much better to override the hierarchy. Indeed there will be occasions on which it is better to ignore even the primary rule, and no further guidance can be offered by the deontological system about when and how to override it.

Should the health service operate according to God-given rules?

It is important to think a little about the sorts of argument people of religious faith might advance in favour of the proposition that the health service should be based on supernatural rules.

Many people base their ethics on what they take to be 'God's law'. At their simplest these personal ethics assume an action is right if it has been divinely approved, and wrong if God has forbidden it. The difficulty facing any plan to base a health service on 'God-given' moral principles is that different people understand 'God's law' differently, and of course many others do not accept there is such a thing at all. Dependent upon which god one recognizes (a major hurdle for a health service based in a multi-religious society), or even dependent upon which sections from religious texts are chosen, different moral principles might be followed.

The problems in this respect are similar to those encountered by rule-deontology:

1 Which of the various laws said to be God-given are truly from a deity? Which are most appropriate for a health service, and which deity will confirm this? And if all divine laws are of equal merit, which should a health service adopt?
2 If all 'divine law' is adopted by health workers then, in the inevitable cases of disagreement, how can health workers resolve conflicts?

There are many compassionate health workers who act according to principles derived from religious conviction. And there are equally caring health workers who act on principles derived from other sources. Well-intentioned principles do not require religious justification. Furthermore, religious justification for behaviour is impossible to sustain without all concerned sharing the faith. Since not all health workers and clients have faith it is neither practical nor necessary to base a health service on God-given rules.

Influence of Immanuel Kant on ethical thinking

Kant's ethics forthrightly places duties above consequences.[79] He wanted to construct an objective ethical theory with its source in human reason. Kant thought that certain principles of behaviour could be discovered by any rational human being because they are part of the human make-up. According to Kant, some principles are moral in themselves. Human beings have the capacity to recognise that some things simply ought to be done.

The categorical imperative

The most important feature of Kant's ethics is known as the 'categorical imperative'. He argued that this imperative is divided into various 'forms', each of which is a duty incumbent upon rational human beings. Kant claimed that any rational human being will be able to see the certainty and necessity of these moral laws by the use of reason.

For present purposes it is not essential to assess all forms of the categorical imperative, or to give a complete account of Kant's argument. However, it is helpful to examine the extent of Kant's emphasis on duties over consequences.

For Kant the only truly moral action is one generated by a pure motive. The truly moral person will do what ought to be done, not after weighing up the pros and cons of what is likely to happen, but simply because she knows she must obey the moral law. Kant wrote:

> To duty every other motive must give place, because duty is a condition of a will good in itself, whose worth transcends everything.[80]

The truly moral act is not influenced by self-interest, nor by consideration of social benefit. The moral person does her duty because she sees she must.

The essence of Kant's categorical imperative

The central principle of the categorical imperative is familiar to several movements, both religious and atheistic, and rests on the belief that human beings are entitled to equal consideration. Although we obviously have different abilities and constantly find ourselves in changing circumstances, we have shared characteristics sufficient to warrant the conclusion that 'we are all in the same boat'. Given this it follows that no moral person will act towards any other person in a way he himself would not wish to be treated, a conclusion encapsulated in Kant's first formulation of the categorical imperative:

Act only on that maxim which you can at the same time will to be universal law.

In other words, act like this only if you wish anyone else in like circumstances to do the same. Before you deliberately say something hurtful, before you steal, before you decide no-one will know you haven't paid your coffee money at work, or before you do nothing when you could have done good, you must genuinely will that your action become universal law.

More specifically, Kant's ethical theory can be divided into three parts. The first is the general dictum discussed briefly above. The second adds more substance to the imperative, and the third part unites the other two:

1 If you wish to act morally act as if your action in each circumstance is to become law for everyone, yourself included, in the future.
2 If you wish to act morally always treat other human beings as 'ends in themselves' and never merely as 'means'. By this Kant meant that it is unethical to treat people as if they are objects – mere tools to be used to further your own ambitions and ends. It is morally essential to recognise that all other people have ends of their own. They have emotions, hopes and anxieties just as you do, and just as you wish to be respected, other people's feelings and aspirations should be respected equally. According to Kant it is fundamentally immoral to exploit a person without considering her an end in her own right.
3 If you wish to act morally always act as a member of a community where all the other members of that community are 'ends', just as you are.

Why did Kant choose these principles?

If you wish to act morally act as if your action in each circumstance is to become law for everyone, yourself included, in the future.

Kant considered it a natural instinct (i.e. a reaction not based upon reason) for people to be self-interested (unless they are enlightened by the 'moral law'). Conversely, the first principle holds that an essential feature of morality is impartiality in the subject. If a person always operates according to the first principle it becomes fundamentally wrong for that person to make an exception of himself. In other words, when considering how to act it is wrong to believe yourself to be of any more merit than anyone else.

The first principle does not state specifically which sorts of action are good or bad. Instead it forces the actor to examine her moral conscience every time she contemplates an action. If she decides she would not like what she is intending to do to someone else to happen to her, or if she will enjoy what she is doing for herself but would not welcome the consequences if everyone behaved in that way, then according to this principle she must conclude that the proposed action is morally wrong.

If you wish to act morally always treat other human beings as 'ends in themselves' and never merely as 'means'.

This principle is intended to add more substance to the first. Kant was not so idealistic as to hope that in each everyday dealing we will consider the wishes and goals of others. It would be bizarre to inquire into the life history of shop assistants met only once, for example. In this case, or in the case of an employer and employee where the relationship depends upon a financial contract, it is inevitable people will treat each other as means. Kant saw nothing wrong with this provided people are not treated always as means. To be moral in an interaction you must respect the other person's ends when appropriate. For example, if the shop assistant breaks down in tears and begs for your help then you should not treat her as a means.

To treat a person 'as an end' is to recognize that the person has his own purposes, just as you have yours. The secret is to imagine your own death. Imagine how much will be lost when you die – a lifetime of hopes, fears, imaginings, achievements and introspection will disappear. A world will expire. Think of other people with this in mind and you can hardly fail to understand what is meant by the advice to treat them as ends. Slavery, for example, is a clear moral wrong according to this way of thinking. When a person is enslaved he is, to quote Aristotle, treated as nothing more than a living tool.

If you wish to act morally always act as a member of a community where all the other members of that community are 'ends', just as you are.

The idea behind Kant's third principle is that a moral agent should act as a member of a community of persons, all of whom are just as able to make moral decisions as the agent herself. The implication of this, and the link with the other two principles, is that each member of the community should respect the desires of others and allow them freedom of decision. Each will recognise that everyone can and should behave as if they, as a result of their choices and actions, are legislating for everyone else.

Politics and ethics

Certain political conclusions follow from Kant's ethical theories. The association between ethics and politics is not always noticed, even though political implications are bound to ensue from any prescriptive ethical theory. The Ethical Grid is part of such a theory, and so has political consequences for health work and the health service. This theory, like Kant's, is a democratic ethic which defines 'a democratic society' as one in which every one of its members can have a say in how it develops. Kantian ethics requires liberty, since each citizen should be as free as possible to choose for herself. It also requires fraternity in the sense that each person should consider himself a member of a moral community – a member of a community shared by others with equal moral rights and responsibilities.

Some problems with Kant's theory of ethics

There is a significant difficulty with Kant's central doctrine:

Act only on that maxim which you can at the same time will to be universal law.

Kant seems to have intended it to cause people to stop to think before acting. A person who wishes to be moral in Kant's sense might, for example, pause before breaking a promise – perhaps a promise to his wife – to consider whether he would wish that the maxim (that it is right for husbands to break promises to their wives) on which he was about to act should become a universal law. Kant was convinced the moral actor would conclude that he could not will this. What would the institution of marriage be like in this case? For Kant, the austere moral philosopher, there could be no exceptions. He could not conceive how any rational person could universalise a maxim that it is right to break promises. Consequently, it followed for Kant that it must always be wrong to break a promise to one's wife.

What are modern health workers to make of Kant's moral philosophy? It might seem that Kant's work can help provide a structured code of practice, allowing each health worker some responsibility for decision-making (since each could imagine herself legislating universally). But this expectation is dashed when one realises the severity of Kant's advice.

His imperatives are unyielding. But in the complex health world the ability to be flexible, to be able to make rapid judgements about complicated ethical problems under pressure, and sometimes to arrive at sensible compromises, is essential to the best health work. A little thought shows it can often be better to make an exception to a moral rule. There are, for instance, occasions when a strong argument can be made that to break a promise to one's wife or husband is the best moral choice. Perhaps you solemnly vowed that if she ever again came home after midnight without letting you know, you would throw her suitcases, clothes, cat and back catalogue of *Harper's and Queen* out the window. And it turns out her car and cell 'phone *truly* have broken down in the wilds.

But Kant's position is relentlessly uncompromising. There can be no exceptions to the duty to keep a promise, to tell the truth, or whatever else the duty is. If it is right to keep a promise in one instance then it must also be right to keep a promise in any other. Moreover, Kant took little account of the consequences of actions. Although he must have believed that doing one's duty causes desirable consequences, this thought seems to have occurred only on an intellectual plane.

It is not difficult to think of exceptions to the sorts of duty Kant imagined should be moral law. Consider the duty to act on the maxim 'tell the truth', which Kant thought the rational person must will. Imagine that a badly injured man regains consciousness in a hospital bed. He is critically ill and fighting for his life after a road accident. It is hard to see how it makes moral sense to tell him the truth – that his wife and three daughters have been killed – until his condition is no longer critical, and the news unlikely to endanger his life (though it would be a different matter if he were about to die).

Consider too the maxim 'minimise harm', where a psychiatrist is considering whether or not to treat compulsorily a woman who has been making intimidating threats. In this case the problem is that it is unclear what the moral legislator would be universalising. In circumstances like this, what counts as harm and which harms are worse than others are matters open to question – so Kant's dictum is not only inflexible but impossible to apply specifically where matters are open to interpretation. The best a legislator might will is that people should act to minimise harm *as they see it*.

Further objections

The earlier part of this book has shown that the nature of ethics is indistinct and disputable, and that there are alternative senses in which morality can be used. Because Kant did not make the difference between morality and immorality exact, it is possible to interpret his general commandments in different ways. In the absence of a practical definition it is possible to offer justifications for behaviour that many theories of ethics would not accept. For instance, a person might will that the maxim 'no-one should steal' should become a universal law, and do so entirely out of self-interest. The person who wills this might have a large house and money in the bank, and be interested only in maintaining this position. Only 'egotism' offers a similar account of morality. Clearly Kant did not intend it, but by leaving the details up to moral agents to decide it seems he must accept this result.

Kant wanted to argue that people should not make deceitful promises, and then break them to suit their own ends. However, even the duty not to make deceitful promises (or not to break promises) is not obviously the most moral course of action in every circumstance. For example, perhaps money has been lent by a corrupt government which tortures dissidents, and the debtor decides to use it to fund a campaign against torture. It would be heartening to be able to agree with Kant that whatever the consequences it is morally important to abide by a pure motive to do one's duty, but such a stance is impossible to prove in this world. Being moral is surely a more complex and burdensome responsibility than sticking to abstract duties. Striving to be moral is difficult – it requires good intentions but also demands thought, foresight, logic, detachment and integrity – human qualities just as precious as the supposed faculty of pure reason.

The principle of ends offers incomplete advice about how to act morally. If a person attempts to adopt the principle of ends in real life he will inevitably be faced with situations where he will affect people whom he will not be able to treat as ends. If, for instance, a scarce resource can be offered only to a proportion of those who could benefit from it, then the actor who is in a position to distribute it, and who wishes to treat all potential recipients as ends, faces an impossible task. She might, for instance, be an admissions tutor at university, and dearly wish to admit all who have applied to her degree course. But places are limited and only some applicants can have their wishes respected, and so be treated as ends. The remainder, no matter how kind the letter of rejection, must be discarded as if they are of no account, just because life is often like that.

If a person fails to treat as ends all those he might have treated as ends, then he has offended against the moral law as Kant perceived it. What is more, the principle of ends offers no criterion by which to decide who should be treated as ends, when not everyone can.

What features should health workers note most of all about Kant's ethical theory?

The core of Kant's moral philosophy is that once a person is in tune with his moral conscience it is a relatively simple matter to act in the most moral way. For Kant moral issues are not complex or insoluble – ethics is not cerebral perpetual motion – rather it is possible for a person to be consistently moral, and moral in exactly the same way as all other persons within the moral community, by using the faculty of reason. Through reflection and introspection it is possible, according to Kant, to discover laws. It is not enough simply to obey rules because it is legal or because it is part of your job (those who carry out immoral instructions from their superiors can have no moral defence for their actions in Kant's view). Personal motive is crucial. It is up to individuals to discover the pure motives (the moral path) for themselves, often in spite of external pressure to the contrary. Health workers who insist on following instructions and codes because it is expedient for them to do so may well find something in Kant's work to move them to revise their opinions.

Universalisability is another feature of Kant's moral philosophy. It is important for health workers to note that this idea rests on the notion that all people are equal in crucial respects, whatever their position and circumstances in life. Consequently, at least according to Kant, it is fundamentally immoral to act towards one person or group of persons in situation X whilst acting differently towards other persons also in situation X, whatever the external justification. What is so impressive about Kant's work is his insistence that all people should be treated as ends acting within a community in which all other people have equal status as moral agents, or potential moral agents, and are entitled to equal respect because of this – whatever their economic status or whatever their age or physical condition. (Actually there were some exceptions. Kant thought criminals should be punished because, through their crimes, they sacrifice the right to be treated as ends – and this part of his argument is inconsistent with the rationale of work for health presented in this book.)

In sum, Kant prizes individual responsibility and believes that people ought to be treated as equals, since we all share the uniquely human ability to reason morally. This fact transcends our material differences. What is perhaps less useful to health workers is his idea that individual responsibility and freedom to make the best moral judgements stops when universalisable rules are discovered. In the fraught world of health care there are cases in which the human interest is best served by suspending 'moral laws'.

Finally, the most significant inadequacy of Kant's theory – an inadequacy health workers ignore at their peril – is its underemphasis on consequences. In the real world it is no defence, either morally or legally, to say that what was done was done out of a pure motive to be moral. Considerations of logic, probability of outcome and actual outcome must enter the picture when the degree of morality is assessed.

A more complete view of morality comes into play when the consequences are considered. The ethical realm incorporates much more than pure motive – just like in law where conspiracy to murder (intent to murder) and actual murder (where the consequence is that life is lost) are different crimes with different punishments. And beyond the legal sphere, wanting to be kind to another person is not the same as actually being kind to her. Actually being kind to a person surely shows a higher degree of morality than meaning to, but never getting around to it.

The ethic of consequences

What is consequentialism and what is utilitarianism?

For the sake of clarity it is important to explain the difference between consequentialism and utilitarianism. Consequentialism is the more global ethical theory, utilitarianism its major subset. Such are the similarities between the two that it is sufficient to introduce consequentialism, and to direct the majority of the discussion to utilitarianism – the best known term.

Consequentialism

On the face of it consequentialism is a straightforward doctrine, apparently diametrically opposed to Kant's version of deontology. In its most radical form consequentialism holds that the rightness or wrongness of an act should be judged solely on whether its consequences produce more benefits than disadvantages, the nature of 'benefit' and 'disadvantage' having been defined beforehand by the consequentialist. A consequentialist decides how to act by assessing the likely outcomes of her proposed action, and judges the morality of what she has or has not done according to how her action turns out.

Utilitarianism

Utilitarianism is classically associated with the goal of happiness or pleasure. However, moral philosophers have come to think such a simple measure rather crude, and other measures of utility are now considered legitimate. Indeed it is now rather artificial to distinguish between utilitarianism and consequentialism.

Unlike deontological theory, utilitarianism does not depend upon principles and commandments – it does not assume that there are naturally right things to do. Utilitarianism is not concerned with motives for actions, but with the results of actions. At its simplest the utilitarian prescription is this: a person ought always to act so as to produce the greatest balance of good over bad.

But what is good and what is bad? The earliest form of utilitarianism defined 'the good' as 'pleasure' or 'happiness'. The 'greatest happiness principle' of Jeremy Bentham (who, along with Mill, is most usually associated with utilitarianism) states that a person should attempt to achieve 'the greatest good, or greatest happiness, of the greatest number' (though this formula does not make it clear whether the good should be distributed as widely and equally as possible or is best concentrated in the hands of a few). One alternative definition of the utilitarian good was proposed by G.E. Moore who thought, presumably on the basis of his own preferences, that the central human goods were personal relationships and aesthetic experiences.[80]

But whatever the definition of good and evil these goods and evils must be *measurable*. It is crucial to utilitarianism (the forebear of economics) that a cost–benefit calculation can be made. A judgement about what to do cannot depend on opinion only; rather it must be possible to work out an answer according to standards laid down beforehand.

Importantly, utilitarianism does not hold that the highest good is the good of the self (which would be a form of egotism) but insists that the person working out what to do (the moral agent) must be considered of equal importance to everyone else in the assessment. As Mill argues:

> The utilitarian standard of what is right in conduct is not the agent's own happiness but that of all considered. As between his own happiness and that of others, utilitarianism requires him to be as strictly impartial as a disinterested and benevolent spectator.[81]

In other words utilitarianism requires that a person should *sacrifice* his self-interest if this is likely to bring about an increase in the general good.

Types of utilitarianism

Act-utilitarianism

Act-utilitarianism states that in any situation a person should, if he is to do the right thing, assess which of the actions open to him is most likely to produce the greatest balance of good over evil (however defined). It falls to the act-utilitarian, in each case he faces, to ask: 'What effect will my action have on the amount of good in the world?' Where a deontologist might think he has a moral duty to keep promises in all circumstances, an act-utilitarian will not take this for granted. Instead, in the light of the unique and specific prevailing conditions, he will weigh up the pros and cons of keeping the promise, always giving the fullest possible attention to a consideration of the likely outcome. If keeping the promise does not seem likely to produce a balance of good over evil then – according to act-utilitarianism – he is justified in breaking it.

Act-utilitarian problem-solving need not be quite as ad hoc as this since act-utilitarians must also access the likely effects (short and long term) on other people, caused by a glib breaking of a promise for the sake of expedience. And it may be that the decrease in general levels of integrity is not a considered price worth paying.

Act-utilitarianism can best be described as a form of opportunism. It does not endorse rules other than the requirement to calculate (although there is a modified form of act-utilitarianism that permits 'rules of thumb' based on past experiences – to avoid having to deliberate afresh every time). If, on balance, the outcome of your intended action is likely to be good, then do it! Do it whatever it is, even if it is stealing, or lying, or causing physical harm, or destroying someone emotionally, or blackmailing, or breaking the law of the land, or murdering someone, or betraying a friend. If you think your action will produce more good than evil in the end, then that is what you should do.

What features of act-utilitarianism are relevant for health workers?

First, it is difficult to imagine any national system suggesting its staff become act-utilitarians. For example, enthusiastic converts might seek to justify a lower standard of care – or even non-voluntary euthanasia – for old people occupying beds that could be used to care for younger people. Such discrimination, although possibly justifiable in utilitarian terms, is not work for health.

There is a further practical problem. The act-utilitarian must assess, in each and every case, the likely ratio of good and evil. Yet this requirement is unrealistic in the urgent health care world. What is needed is a way of reflection that does not demand calculation afresh in every case, yet which nevertheless offers individuals the opportunity to think for themselves.

This focus on individual responsibility is the main advantage of act-utilitarianism. Just as act-deontology claims that a person has a basic duty to reflect on the array of principles available, so act-utilitarianism offers a compelling reminder that inherited rules of practice need not be obeyed in all cases. Given rules might be disobeyed if the health worker calculates it is better to do so. Sometimes sticking to the rules might produce unacceptable consequences (perhaps the house rule is to offer only cursory explanations of treatment, and never to offer additional information once the consultant has said his piece).

General utilitarianism

This version of utilitarianism advocates neither unique responses nor rules. Instead, general utilitarianism requires a potential actor to ask, 'What if everyone were to do what I propose to do?' For example, a doctor of medicine about to deceive a patient about his condition should ask himself what the consequences would be if everyone hid information they think other people do not want to hear.

General utilitarianism is uncomplicated. Most people have said disapprovingly, 'What if everybody did that?' and there is worth in this common dictum. However, as far as health care is concerned the theory is a little incomplete, and is best used as a stimulus to thought. For instance, recall the case of Diane the health visitor (see **Chapter Three**), whose aim was not to produce the highest possible proportion of child immunisations, but to enable parents to weigh up the pros and cons of vaccinating their children. For Diane the highest priority was not a possible decrease in disease and illness, but a possible increase in the level of education. The response to Diane, 'But what if everyone did that?', is commonplace amongst community nurses who argue, for instance, that if all health visitors saw themselves as remedial educators rather than medical workers this might have bad consequences for the health service, whose level of future funding depends in part upon the sort of 'performance indicator' good immunisation rates produce. And how would general practitioners react to an army of rebel 'nurse educators'?

However, 'what if everybody did that?' is not always a damning response. It is equally possible for nurses who think like Diane to ask 'what if everybody did that' of those who think of immunisation work as a 'sales campaign'.

Rule-utilitarianism

Echoing rule-deontology, rule-utilitarianism argues that personal judgement, not obedience to rules, is fundamental to morality. But where rule-deontology applies pre-ordained rules, rule-utilitarianism holds that rules of conduct are to be worked out by discovering which, if always adhered to, will produce the greatest balance of good over evil. The justification for rules is in their utility rather than their purity, but this proviso apart, there are marked similarities between rule-deontology and rule-utilitarianism.

In contrast to act-utilitarianism, where it can be acceptable to maintain rules – but only as a general guideline – a rule-utilitarian wants to keep a rule that will produce the greatest good in the long run. So, for example, a rule-utilitarian might calculate that the best consequences result from obedience to the rule 'always tell the truth'.

The difference between act-utilitarianism and rule-utilitarianism can be demonstrated like this.

You are a health education officer. You are aware that your friend has been stealing from the stationery store regularly for the last 2 years. Most people you know have done something like this in the past, and it is not usually regarded as a serious crime. It is seen more as a perk of the job. However, one day your manager asks you a direct question, 'Has Albert stolen the coloured duplicating paper meant for those posters to publicise our "learning communities for a holistic 2010" meeting?' You know he has and you know also that if you tell the truth your friend's job will be in serious danger.

It is likely, although of course not certain, that an act-utilitarian would say utility demands that a lie be told to help Albert and his family – after all it is only a minor misdemeanour and will perhaps be the jolt he needs to stop – while a rule-utilitarian would tell the truth on the ground that it is better in the long run, even though there might be temporary benefit in telling a lie.

What features of rule-utilitarians are relevant for health workers?

Rule-utilitarian health workers use rules derived from careful consideration of past costs and benefits. Their principal problem is a difficulty for all varieties of utilitarianism (including health economics). That is, there may be occasions on which their policy creates an excess of good over evil for a population as a whole, but does not distribute it fairly. Thus a principle of justice (that all social goods ought to be distributed equally) is undermined by utilitarianism. The British Labour Party argued that just such a calculation was made by the Tory Government of the 1980s. There is considerable utility in maintaining a high level of unemployment (unions are kept under control because there is endemic fear of unemployment, output increases, house costs decrease and there is an increase in the standard of living for those in permanent, well-paid jobs). The majority enjoy benefit (and so are more likely to vote for you next time) while the minority suffer, and on utilitarian terms this is fair enough.

To take a health service example, it might promote utility to move non-dangerous mentally ill people from hospitals to the community. It might save money and it might help some patients become happier and better adjusted, but if such a policy were carried out without room for exceptions then there would inevitably be some patients, relatives and carers who suffer (many mental health workers and consumers say this actually has been the effect of over-zealous de-institutionalisation in recent years).

Here is a classic illustration of utilitarianism's clash with justice as fairness:

> Let us imagine that the happiness of the whole human race were to be immeasurably increased – poverty eliminated, brotherhood achieved, disease conquered . . . but the condition is that one man, his life mysteriously prolonged, is to be kept involuntarily in a state of continuous and agonising torture. According to the utilitarian criterion, which measures the rightness of an act by its results, it would seem that the argument is justified . . . the net balance of the utilitarian moral scale would have to point in the direction of maximum happiness and away from the eternal agony of the single suffering man. But most people who consider the proposed bargain feel that there is something terribly wrong with it.[82]

A further general problem with utilitarianism arises because utilitarians must claim that any action is right so long as it brings about favourable consequences – even if the intention of the actor was clearly evil. For example, imagine that through deliberate and excessive cost-cutting a private cosmetic surgeon has disfigured 50 patients, two of whom were driven to suicide as a result. The malpractice comes to light and the doctor is struck off the medical register, compensation paid to all victims and – most important of all – a thorough policing of cosmetic surgery advertisers is carried out in future. This ensures such malpractice cannot reoccur, thus sparing potentially thousands of people unnecessary trauma. Since this is the outcome the utilitarian must define the corrupt doctor's actions moral, despite his immoral intent.

To give an example beyond the medical field, in 1996 Martyn Bryant went on a crazy rampage in Port Arthur in Tasmania, killing 35 people and seriously damaging the lives of thousands of their friends and relatives. Bryant's intent cannot possibly be described as moral yet, because Australia's gun laws (and those of some other countries) have been stiffened up and police monitoring of dangerous people made more rigorous, his actions will probably increase happiness in the long-term. Such incongruities as these are hard to reconcile unless utilitarians are prepared to dilute their ideas with aspects of other moral theories. But if they do this then their approaches can no longer be described as utilitarian.

(Note: it would be wrong to think of deontologists and consequentialists as tribespeople, always acting in accord with the dictates of their preferred moral theory. In reality those who espouse technical ethics treat the subject like a game. For the sake of argument or prestige a philosopher will sometimes defend a position to the hilt – for instance, she might argue that in every possible circumstance her idiosyncratic version of rule-utilitarianism is always the most moral option – but rarely, if ever, will she carry this position into everyday life.)

The four principles approach

Two decades ago two American academics, Tom Beauchamp and Jim Childress, published the 'four principles approach' to medical ethics.[83–86] This idea has proved widely influential in both teaching and writing about medical ethics, particularly amongst clinicians and nurses with little or no philosophical knowledge. I have lost count of the papers I have read that state – almost always without argument or elucidation – that 'the four principles of medical/health care/bioethics are beneficence, non-maleficence, respect for autonomy and justice'.

Beachamp describes the principles more fully as:

1 Beneficence (the obligation to provide benefits and balance benefits against risks)
2 Non-maleficence (the obligation to avoid the causation of harm)
3 Respect for autonomy (the obligation to respect the decision-making capacities of autonomous persons)
4 Justice (obligations of fairness in the distribution of benefits and risks).[83]

The four principles idea is deceptively simple. By using these principles, either singly or in combination, a doctor is supposed to be able to give a satisfactory answer to any moral problem he comes across in his work. He may need 'additional interpretation and specification' and further rules such as 'Don't kill' and 'Tell the truth', but the four principles are thought by their advocates to provide an adequate framework for all moral deliberation in health care.

Raanan Gillon, past editor of the *Journal of Medical Ethics* and a four principles devotee, offers fulsome support of Beauchamp and Childress:

> In brief, the four principles plus scope approach claims that whatever your personal philosophy, politics, religion, moral theory or life stance, you will find no difficulty in committing yourself to four *prima facie* moral principles plus a concern for their scope of application . . . these . . . can be seen to encompass most if not all of the moral issues that arise in health care (I am increasingly inclined to believe that the approach can, if sympathetically interpreted, be seen to encompass *all* moral issues, not merely those arising in health care). . . . 'Prima facie' . . . means that the principle is binding unless it conflicts with another moral principles – if it does then you have to choose between them. The four principles approach does not claim to provide a method for doing so. . . . [W]hat the principles . . . approach *can* provide is a common set of moral commitments, a common moral language, and a common set of moral issues to be considered in particular cases, before coming to your own answer, using your preferred moral theory or other approach to choosing between these principles when they conflict.[85]

Beauchamp affirms Gillon's understanding of prima facie:

> [The four principles] . . . are *prima facie*: they are always binding *unless* they conflict with obligations expressed in another moral principle, in which case a balancing of the demands of the two principles is necessary. In this event, further specification is required of the precise commitments of the guidelines for the special circumstance(s). Which principle overrides in a case of conflict will depend on the particular context, which is likely to have unique features.[83]

Beauchamp admits that:

> Some have severely criticised the four-principles approach as a 'mantra of principles', meaning that the principles have functioned for some adherents like a ritual incantation of norms repeated with little reflection or analysis[83]

and cites three criticisms in particular:

> Gert and Clouser bring the following accusations . . . (1) the 'principles' are little more than checklists or headings for lists of values worth remembering, and so the principles have no deep moral substance and do not produce directive guidelines for moral conduct; (2) principles analyses fail to provide a theory of justification or a theory that ties the principles together so as to generate clear, coherent, specific rules, with the consequence that the principles and so-called derivative rules are *ad hoc* constructions without systematic order; (3) these *prima facie* principles must often compete in difficult circumstances, yet the underlying account is unable to decide how to adjudicate the conflict in particular cases and unable theoretically to deal with a conflict of principles.[83]

Astonishingly, Beauchamp not only does not deny that these are problems, but is quite unable to offer any answer to them. His only defence is that they are also problems for anyone else who uses principles or rules. He then uses a dismally ubiquitous academic's ploy – he is unable to fortify his own position so he attacks his critics' thinking instead.

The four principles approach is manifestly empty, and has achieved its great popularity as a direct result. Because the principles lack detail – and since their adherents' attempted justifications swiftly collapse into waffle – they can be used by almost anyone to defend almost anything, and have a special appeal to those for whom existing arrangements are good. For such lucky men and women the principles will very likely seem to:

> Encompass most if not all of the moral issues that arise in health care (and may) be seen to encompass *all* moral issues[85]

because they will rarely if ever have reason to question them:

> In this event, further specification is required of the precise commitments of the guidelines for the special circumstance(s). Which principle overrides in a case of conflict will depend on the particular context, which is likely to have unique features.[83]

Gillon and Beauchamp's use of *'prima facie'* is inescapably authoritarian. Here is Gillon's version again:

> Whatever your personal philosophy, politics, religion, moral theory or life stance, you will find no difficulty in committing yourself to four *prima facie* moral principles plus a concern for their scope of application . . . these . . . can be seen to encompass most if not all the moral issues that arise in health care. . . . *'Prima facie'* . . . means that the principle is binding unless it conflicts with another moral principle – if it does then you have to choose between them. The four principles approach does not claim to provide a method for doing so.[85]

Let's look at this a little more closely. We are asked to accept – no, we are told – that each of the four principles is objectively binding on us – only if there are conflicts can a principle be disregarded, and then only if it is overridden by one of the other three. The ethical question is thus never – do I accept the social arrangements which generated this ethical problem (not enough money for care of the elderly, for instance)? – and always – which moral truth should I bring to bear to offer the best solution in the circumstances I accept as given?

Gillon's claim is so astounding it is hard to believe it has been taken seriously:

> Whatever your personal philosophy, politics, religion, moral theory or life stance, you will find no difficulty in committing yourself to four *prima facie* moral principles plus a concern for their scope of application.[85]

As a matter of fact this is nonsense. If you are a Marxist, or a Sartrian, or a utilitarian, or a different sort of deontologist, or a cultural relativist (to name but a few) you will have an insurmountable difficulty accepting the four principles because they will not be part of the moral theory you espouse.

Gert and Clouser's criticisms are, of course, spot on. In addition, each of the principles is open to interpretation so wide that it is unintelligible to state 'I am following principle

X' without further explanation of what you take X to mean. And if you do bother to spell out what you mean more exactly you will find you have gone beyond the principles anyway – intelligent reflection on moral priorities renders the four principles redundant.

But the worst problem with the four principles approach is that it does not explain *why* one should follow it. Of course it is a helpful teaching tool and can be a useful starting point for analysis, but its proponents never say why respect for autonomy, for instance, should be binding (either in health care or in life in general). It is not self-evident that it should. Indeed in many areas of our lives our autonomy is not respected – and not just in those areas (like road traffic law) where we might harm others (I'd like better wages, my MP to represent my views not his, and all doctors to act on my philosophy, but it doesn't happen). In order to explain why one should choose the four principles matters of meaning and purpose have to be addressed – philosophical questions must be determinedly pursued in order to develop an underlying theory capable of supporting moral conclusions.

Beauchamp, Childress and Gillon have got it lamentably wrong. Nebulous principles generally acceptable to well-heeled Western liberals do no more than offer conclusions: (a) open to wide interpretation; and (b) acceptable only to those who agree with them in the first place ('justice' is a prime example, and is discussed in the following section). In order to engage in serious moral reflection it is necessary first to have a sustained and specific understanding of the importance of your enterprise. This way there can be constructive disagreement with those who hold alternative theories, key words such as 'autonomy' and 'justice' will have clear and distinctive meaning, and there will be no need for the hopeless assumption that everyone is bound by obviously contestable ideas. Given strong theories of purpose controversy can take place where it ought to – over the meaning and importance of practical health and social goals.

Are these criticisms too harsh?

From time to time, but not for long, I wonder if I am being unfair to the 'principalists'. However, I find that all I need to do to assure myself that I am after all being perfectly reasonable is briefly to dip into Beauchamp and Childress at random, reacquainting myself with their simplistic generalisations. For example, I found this gem within 2 minutes:

> Since virtually everyone grows up with a basic understanding of the institution of morality, its norms are readily understood. All persons who are serious about living a moral life already grasp the core dimensions of morality. They know not to lie, not to steal property, to keep promises, to respect the rights of others, not to kill or cause harm to innocent persons, and the like.[86]

It is utter nonsense. There can be good reasons to lie and to steal and even to cause harm to 'innocent persons' (see the discussion of utilitarianism above), as every intelligent person understands from life experience.

I am by no means the only person to despair at the influence such poor thinking continues to have on the training of health professionals:

Too often, bioethicists exaggerate their capacity to bring longstanding ethical debates to ultimate closure. They mistakenly claim that morality is settled, orderly, and in a state of reflective equilibrium when this account tells only one part of a very complex story. In pluralistic societies, we find both relatively stable social norms as well as conflicting understandings of how we should live and die. Several of the dominant approaches in bioethics rely upon the notion of shared, common, intuitively obvious moral norms. However, many of the issues addressed by bioethicists reveal the existence of disagreements over what constitutes 'common sense' moral reasoning. Disputes about ethical issues in medicine, healthcare and biotechnology often occur along cultural and religious fault lines. Such conflicts emerge in clinical settings, the deliberations of advisory bodies and professional organizations, and in legislative arenas.[87]

Justice

What is justice?

This question is as difficult as 'what is health?' The only certainty is that a definitive answer is impossible. As with 'health' there are several meaningful uses of the word, all of which are sometimes claimed as the true meaning. However, none of them should be allowed to dominate because it is only in multiplicity that the richest sense of justice can be gleaned.

Justice is commonly thought of in two ways: justice as fairness and justice as appropriate punishment for wrongdoing. Justice as fairness is violated when people equal in all relevant aspects are nevertheless treated unequally. Justice as appropriate punishment for wrongdoing is known as retributive justice, but this aspect is not of concern in the present inquiry.

Three versions of justice as fairness

Justice as fairness can be subdivided in three interesting ways – all of which are undoubtedly part of the notion of justice overall, but only one of which is fundamental to a true health service. The three types are: to each according to his rights, to each according to what he deserves, and to each according to his need. Of these, only the final dictum informs the richest sense of work for health.[88]

The expression 'to each according to his rights' is essentially contractual justice. For example, if a person agrees to labour for a specified sum of money it is his right – and it is just – that his employer pays him his due (so long as the worker has abided by the conditions of the contract). The phrase 'to each according to what he deserves' is used to justify meritocracies, in which those who work the hardest or most successfully gain the best rewards. If a woman puts in long hours building up a business then, if there is to be justice in this sense, she should reap the harvest of her endeavours. Similarly, if a man strives diligently to obtain a good university degree, accruing debt and sacrificing the opportunity to earn more outside university then – according to his understanding of justice – it is only fair that he should eventually be accorded the status and earning power that his studying and application merit.

Both these concepts are highly contentious. For example, in Western countries people have equal rights to own property, but some people are hugely rich while others have nothing. These inequalities are so marked that it might be argued that an alternative principle of justice (usually 'to each according to need') should override 'to each according to his right', at least in exceptional cases. Likewise with justice as desert, which is called into question by considerations such as this: perhaps the young man who has worked hard at university does in a sense deserve to enjoy the benefits of his dedication. But this is tempered by the knowledge that he has been privileged to have been able to attend a good university in the first place. Not everyone can secure a university place – and far fewer are able to find a place at a decent institution. Because they enjoy a sound upbringing – which brings early access to books, a wide parental vocabulary and positive peer pressures – middle-class children have a better chance of attending a good university than their working-class contemporaries, even though their talents might be equivalent.

Of course the above discussion is superficial, and it may also be argued that justice as 'to each according to his need' has inadequacies at least as serious. However, this book maintains that this should be a founding principle of a true health service. Indeed it is already embraced by health workers who wish to help anybody overcome physical and mental problems – whoever they are and whatever they have done.

True work for health is not driven primarily by the wish to ensure that contracts are honoured (although this is sometimes important), nor does it cater only to those considered to have earned it; rather it concentrates first and foremost on people's needs[8] whether these are food, or warmth, or shelter, or surgery, or kindness, or advice, or education, or love. True health care is informed by a notion of justice that regards the fulfilment of need, equally and without unwarranted discrimination, as a fundamental premise.

A developed notion of justice – Rawls and 'justice as fairness'

Although the idea of justice cannot be given a full analysis in this book, it is such a central notion in health work that it is worth introducing the work of John Rawls, a modern philosopher influential in this area. Rawls worked out an elaborate system by which to ensure a just social organisation,[89] or so he thought.

The just society arising from a veil of ignorance

Rawls's theory is complicated but insists fundamentally that the unequal possession and distribution of such desired qualities as power, wealth and income is unjust unless these inequalities work to benefit the worst-off citizens.

In order to demonstrate the strength of this claim Rawls asks us to imagine ourselves in a hypothetical situation, in which we are a free, logical, yet disinterested being about to enter into a social contract with everyone else. The most intriguing feature of Rawls's proposal is that none of the parties to the contract knows what or where they will be in the society when it has taken shape. The contract is to be made behind a veil of ignorance which conceals completely the actual place and condition of all involved. The contractor might be male or female, young or old, employer or employee, rich or poor, diseased or not.

After asking us to imagine this pre-contractual situation Rawls asks: which principles should govern social arrangements behind the veil? In other words, which principles inform the just society?

It is well worth reflecting on Rawls's challenge, since in one way or another all moral matters are shaped by social structure and organisation. Rawls's own answer (but not the only one) is this.

There should be two main principles of social justice, and the first should take precedence over the second where they conflict:

1 Each person should have an equal right to the maximum amount of liberty consistent with a similar liberty for others. In other words, each person should have as much freedom as possible unless or until this freedom works against the freedoms of other people. The basic liberties, according to Rawls, are political liberty, the right to property, freedom from arbitrary arrest, and to be within a system of law that deals impartially with all who come under its rule.
2 Any social and economic inequalities should be organised so that they work to everyone's advantage, including the worst-off. In a modern and complex society, which is bound to contain people of different abilities, there will inevitably be some inequalities. But if these inequalities work only for the benefit of those already privileged then they should not be allowed. An example of a justifiable inequality, on Rawls's account, is for a surgeon to be well-off, but only because his skills have the potential to contribute to the well-being of all. Societies without the services of the rich surgeons will be worse off, Rawls thinks.

Like any argument in political philosophy, Rawls's position is open to criticism. It has, for example, been argued that Rawls's response is by no means the only feasible conclusion that might be reached from behind the veil. Why, for instance, did Rawls prefer liberty above equality? There is no reason to think that some social contractors behind the veil of ignorance would not conclude that the best way of ensuring justice within a society is to guarantee equal distribution of resources, even at the cost of a lower level of personal liberty in the populace. After all, we are not asked to imagine contractors already living in a liberal social regime, but people whose political outlooks are entirely unpolluted by experience and education. Indeed, Rawls's own judgement does not appear to have been made in total ignorance, but is informed by prior adherence to liberal ideals. He assumes that the 'rational person' behind the veil of ignorance is 'rational' in a particular way. Regardless of the actual identity of surgeons, and dustmen, the ignorant 'rationalist' is supposed to think it right a priori that such grossly unequal roles and status should exist in a just society. Rawls cannot think that social structures different from those that currently make up Western society will be entertained for long. He does not envisage any person behind the veil prepared to argue for absolute equality of education for fear that he might then be at risk through the absence of trained surgeons.

But of course it is by no means absurd to think that some contractors might be prepared to bargain for a system of education that does not stream and create elite specialisms. It is not out of the question that a different system of education could eliminate the need for so many surgeons, nor is it necessarily the case that a more egalitarian system of education, and even more equal later financial reward, will result in a scarcity of trained surgeons (people might just decide to become surgeons for the challenge and job satisfaction).

The pros and cons of Rawls's theory of justice are not a major concern for this inquiry, however. But what is central is the powerful connection between politics and morality, which Rawls's work serves to highlight. The political structure of a society is profoundly and intimately linked to the level of morality that exists. If social structures enable some people to achieve worthwhile potentials but do not allow others equivalent chances – then morality is not being created as fully as it should be (in my opinion). In the concluding chapters of this book it is argued that since work for health is a moral endeavour, and that since health care is to act justly, then the entire performance of the health service – its administration, its hierarchies, its priorities and its resourcing – is of moral concern because it is directly and constantly responsible for creating or diminishing the degree of morality in the world.

Summary

Chapter Six has given a basic account of two classic approaches to moral reasoning: deontology and consequentialism. This, together with **Chapter Four's** discussion of the foundation of morality, should provide health workers with sufficient background and working material to begin to reflect with at least some confidence about technical morality in health care. It also serves as essential preparation for understanding and using the Ethical Grid.

Obstacles to Clear Moral Reasoning

Introduction

Chapter Seven lists two different ways in which moral reasoning can be polluted. 'Bad faith' corrupts moral reasoning as people come to believe that they have to think in certain conventional ways, and have to uphold professional values, even if they do not hold these values as individuals, deep down. While health economics – and QALYs and their derivatives especially[90] – corrupts moral reasoning with the claim that personal judgements are ultimately irrelevant, however deeply held they are, since cost calculations are always the deciding factor in health service decision-making.

It would be possible to add many other obstacles to moral reasoning to this chapter – for example, human beings' sheep-like integrative tendencies; universities that try to tell students what to think; and news media that try to discourage everybody from thinking at all – but the point to emphasise is a positive one: that though there is no objective morality, moral reasoning is a profoundly honest, personal, partly introspective exploration of one's commitment to life. This exploration can include professional considerations and roles, and it can also incorporate cost–benefit calculations and matters of evidence – but these should never be the only factors and should never obscure the essential values-based elements.

Bad faith

Honesty and integrity are essential in moral reasoning. One way to reveal their importance is to contemplate 'bad faith'.

According to Jean-Paul Sartre, people guilty of bad faith fail to be true to themselves – they deny their individuality and freedom by burying it in a role.[91] Unfortunately, playing out a predefined role is a characteristic commonly displayed by people who become professionals. As we have seen, when some people become 'professional' they seem to change – sometimes quite radically – from how they were before. Their very identities appear to alter to fit the position taken on. Some become so addicted they imagine 'professional moral responsibility' is different from 'personal moral responsibility', and become morally lost as a result (the soldier blindly carrying out orders, the surgeon who thinks his job is only to cut and stitch, the lawyer happy to have persuaded a jury to acquit her guilty client – each exhibit this tendency).

Sartre saw that we must all cope with an irrational world – a world, despite superficial appearances, without order and structure. In this random universe things just happen and we have no real control over them. Nothing is determined. Events are free and conform to no pattern. Our canons of rationality, logic, order and coherence are only a facade. Reality is chaotic and meaningless. We categorise the world, and we categorise ourselves. We must, for if we did not we would feel permanently disorientated – forever anguished and nauseous. However, by creating a comforting, artificial world we lose touch with what is truly real, and forget our true nature.

Bad faith results from habitual denial of this truth. Once we see ourselves as bound to act in a certain way, once we say 'I have no choice in this matter', then we have deceived ourselves and are acting in bad faith. Bad faith is the failure to realise that any role has originally been a matter of choice, and that it remains a matter of choice whether to continue to perform it or not.

Bad faith is exhibited, for example, when a person buys a luxury item – perhaps a watch with a plain granite face which makes telling the time a matter of guesswork – and justifies the purchase by saying it was essential. There are many who see themselves as a stereotype – as the dutiful housewife with two children, cooking meals at set times for her husband, just as her mother did before her; or as the kindly paternalistic general practitioner; or as the angry, certain, righteous member of Militant; or as the total feminist; or as the idle erudite philosopher sponging a good wage from the State, always 'writing a book' but never finishing it. These people's tastes, beliefs and actions are dictated not by themselves but by the roles they play.

Sartre thought that the man who exhibits bad faith is striving to become an object, sacrificing creativity for the security of a tried and trusted role. The man with bad faith tries to become an object in order to lose true consciousness, and as a result abdicates responsibility. He throws away choice for the sake of becoming a pawn. Bad faith is a personal disgrace, for where there is no real choice there can be no moral development. For Sartre, no matter what the rules, there is always choice. Not to recognise this is to ossify – which is the worst crime a person can commit against himself.

Although Sartre's philosophy may be difficult to accept – and this book certainly does not argue that health professionals should act as if the world is utterly chaotic – his insight is illuminating and has ramifications for moral action.

Essence and existence – an expansion

This book's central questions are: what are human beings for? What is it about us that makes our existence truly worthwhile, and what is it that degrades us? Of course these are not matters that can be finally proved, but they should be constantly discussed. Sartre's contribution is important in two ways. First, he reminds us of the presence of our remarkable capacity for free choice. He then shows that the existence of this capacity has implications for the way societies and their institutions are arranged.

Sartre drew a fundamental distinction between people and objects. Objects – chairs, satchels or beer mugs, for instance – have an essence. What they are is predetermined, their nature fixed according to their given function. But people are not like this. We do not have an allotted essence or 'shape' as objects do. People simply have existence, a fact that allows unadulterated freedom to create oneself uniquely. So much freedom is so frightening that many of us feel unable to face up to it, preferring to think of ourselves as essences instead.

Satre's idea is as naive as it is penetrating. It takes no account of genetics, for instance, and fails to appreciate that no-one has infinite potential. Nor does it recognise how greatly people can be constrained by external circumstances and events (as Sartre was to realise later in his life). But despite these considerable oversights, Sartre's moral ideal is enormously important.

A further problem

It is a fact of life that very many of us are content to be instructed. Not everyone wants to take responsibility, and not everyone is inclined to take creative risks. Some people insist there is much they would rather not know, even about their medical treatment. Some of us do not want autonomy (Understanding B – see **Chapter Nine**) because it is taxing, and it can hurt. Most of us are trusting, submissive and happy to have our horizons defined for us. Why should people not spend their lives in cotton wool if that is what they wish? Why should people not freely decide to abdicate their autonomy in favour of being looked after by the State, an institution or another person?

In answer, there are two reasons why personal deliberation and independent choosing should be encouraged in all forms of human life, including professional life. First, a person trained habitually to follow given rules is underdeveloped. A vital part of her is left barren when it could be verdant. In extreme cases such a person will have difficulty making any social choices coherently. Even when someone operates under a system of rules there is still need for some deliberation. Is this a situation of the kind in which I should apply this rule? In this case, is this procedure justified? Which of the rules I could use should I choose just now? Second, such a person is not properly equipped to deal with unexpected life circumstances – precisely the situations health workers often face. The rare case, the novel issue (perhaps raised by advances in medical technology), the urgent problem when there is no time to consult the rule book or a superior – all these occur repeatedly. Only someone who has developed his capacity to judge can act thoughtfully – committed rule-followers must stand helplessly by, redundant without their guide. Those who think for themselves are in an infinitely better position. They can follow rules if they believe it wise to do so, and they can override them if they think they should.

An illustration

It is not so difficult to imagine what it is like to throw off the shackles of bad faith. There is an enlightening illustration of the dizziness, the sense of being a stranger in a foreign land, the freedom and the fear, which people can experience when they first try to shake off their bad faith. Yet this illustration is so mundane, and the step so small.

When driving road vehicles it is the law that we must stop at traffic lights on the signal red. In order to avoid accidents and ensure the traffic flows smoothly it can – obviously – be important to obey this particular rule. Occasionally, traffic lights fail and we have to make our own judgement about whether or not it is safe to proceed. So it is for the best that we can choose to disobey faulty signals if we need to. But this is not the most interesting case. Sometimes we are not sure if the traffic lights are working properly. Perhaps it is late at night, there is little traffic and the lights seem to have been on red for a very long time. The rule-follower's car is four cars away from the front of the queue. Then, hesitantly, the leading car begins to move forward despite the red light. It moves away and, again hesitantly, the next car follows, and then the third. What is the committed rule-follower to do?

Once he decides to move it will be like a revelation. Almost magically the rules will melt away, the silly red traffic light will become metal and glass and electrics. The rules will be seen as temporary, man-made, expedient and of minor importance. The rule is not necessary at all, even though it is usually useful. It can be superseded by human judgement. The rule-follower will have been given a glimpse of what it feels like to begin to lose bad faith.

It might be argued that bad faith is a fanciful idea. One has only to observe how many people accept so many social rules without question. Indeed, many people do not even understand that questions are possible. In Britain, for instance, most people accept that the British version of democracy is the only true democracy (despite the existence of several alternative systems around the world), that education for most children should cease at the age of 16, and countless other traditions too. It seems to most people that these things have always been part of British life, and so they assume there can be no other way.

However, just as the belief that things in Britain have always been more or less as they are now is false, so it is also a myth that most people can act only on pre-given rules. Anyone who employs moral reasoning properly – weighing and balancing rules, duties and consequences in order to obtain the best possible outcome – transcends what has been given to her. And all competent people surely have this ability – it is there if we want to use it.

It is also wrong to believe that most of us are unable to recognise the absurd and transient nature of the world. Happily not everyone is an existentialist of Sartre's calibre but people do become aware of the fragility of existence, and the impermanence of even the most precious aspects of life. Because of this it is both right and practical to say: 'Here is a tool – it is not something that can give you certain answers because, as with so much in life, nothing is certain in the moral realm. But it is something that can help you use your judgement.'

None of this is provable, of course. If it is not true that we possess the ability to think for ourselves – or if we are deluded when we believe we are thinking freely – then it is probably a waste of time to provide a general tool to enhance ethical deliberation. But it is at least plausible that the ability to see beyond convention and apparent order is a part of our intellectual make-up. All people, unless they die at an early age, sooner or later become aware that familiar 'certainties' can fall away. They vanish when a person is suddenly made redundant after long service, when parents divorce, and when someone close dies or leaves. These and countless other crises force the recognition that the existence we have come to feel safe with is actually acutely brittle. People with no ability to see this are extremely unusual. For instance, if a parent suffers the death of a child at Christmas then the trimmings, bonhomie and tinsel will appear alien, superficial and unreal. If they do not – even if only temporarily – then this would concern a health worker who wished to facilitate the grieving process, and may well indicate severe psychological disorder.

A further obstacle to clear moral reasoning. QALYs: the wrong kind of cost–benefit analysis

It is easiest to measure those things that can be measured most easily.[10] But it is not always true that the most measurable things are the most valuable:

> It is the mark of the educated man and a proof of his culture that in every subject he looks for only so much precision as nature permits.[59]

Can QALYs be a tool for a health service?

QALYs is an acronym for quality adjusted life years, and 'the QALY' a measure intended to enable the efficient calculation of health service priorities. The QALY is the most well-known tool of health economics, and embodies all that is wrong with this one-eyed approach to policy-making.[90,92–94] In common with other forms of consequentialism QALYs are controversial, though the nature of the controversy is not always clear because the continuing debate tends to generate different sorts of question. Different people expect – and fear – different things from QALYs. Health economists, managers with fixed budgets, doctors facing torturous choices and moral philosophers reflecting at a safe distance, each focus on their most familiar aspects. The economist wants to improve the QALY – so as to make it a more reliable measure; the doctor wonders whether QALYs can help her make efficient decisions; the manager wants to use them to make implicit priorities more explicit; while the philosopher worries about their morality.

What is a QALY?

In the words of Alan Williams, one of the founders of the QALY idea:

> The essence of a QALY is that it takes a year of healthy life expectancy to be worth 1, but regards a year of unhealthy life expectancy as worth less than 1. Its precise value is lower the worse the quality of life of the unhealthy person (which is what the 'quality adjusted' bit is all about). If being dead is worth zero, it is, in principle, possible for a QALY to be negative, i.e. for the quality of a person's life to be judged worse than being dead.

The general idea is that a beneficial health care activity is one that generates a positive amount of QALYs, and that an efficient health care activity is one where the cost per QALY is as low as it can be. A high priority health care activity is one where the cost-per-QALY is low, and a low priority activity is one where the cost-per-QALY is high.[95]

Practically speaking the QALY is a way to assess differences in the quality of life of different individuals. The results it produces are meant to be used in situations where resources are scarce. And it is this application – the use of the QALY to justify rationing – that causes the trouble.

Some critics argue that QALYs are an attempt to dress up discrimination against the sick, elderly and non-productive in pseudo-technical language. Amongst much else, they say the QALY fudges a vital distinction between *quality* of life and the *value* of life, assuming that if a life's quality decreases then its value must drop proportionately. This, it is argued, is an insidious mistake, illustrated by the following *non sequitur*:

1 More 'health output' (or more QALYs – if one accepts the crude definition of health put forward by some health economists)[90] is achieved by spending the same amount of money on Fred as on John.
2 Better cost-effectiveness is obtained by treating Fred rather than John.
3 Therefore Fred's life has more value than John's.

But the value of life is not what it costs to maintain it. If one makes an alternative distinction – between basic 'persons' and 'full persons', for example – then there are good reasons for not confusing value with cost. Although full persons have myriad talents, all people have basic capacities which imply a fundamental equality. There may be huge differences in the quality of their lives – but there can be no differences in the value of their lives seen this way. Just as the criminal law makes no distinction between the murder of a 1-year-old and the murder of an adult, personal existence is equally valuable whether one is 2, 15 or 90. The QALY – on the other hand – assumes the value of human life is not morally fixed but is a 'variable' that can change according to a person's age, ability and social status.

How are QALYs meant to be used?

QALYs may be used for different purposes. They might be employed to decide which of a range of treatments open to a patient will bring about the most favourable quality of life – an ethically inoffensive use, to most people. Alternatively they might be used to discriminate between patients in competition for a scarce resource – an ethically troublesome use.

There are other modes lying between these extremes. QALYs can be deployed in the following ways:

1 To clarify costs of treatment, without generating practical change.
2 To make priorities explicit, so encouraging more self-conscious and rigorous thinking.

3 To compare and assess treatments that produce short-term benefit against those that produce benefit in the long term.

4 To ensure the most cost-effective use of health service funds. For example, hip replacement operations are said to be more cost-effective in QALY terminology than heart transplants. It was noted that studies at York University had come to the conclusion that heart transplants cost over £5000 per QALY compared with £1000 for coronary by-passes and £750 for hip replacements.[96] Since health service funding is finite it was concluded that it is better to channel available funds into hip replacement operations.

5 To ensure the most beneficial distribution, in utilitarian terms, of any available scarce resource – renal dialysis or a drug in short supply, for example.

6 To select for treatment those people who might be expected to produce the most QALYs. Such selection is reminiscent of the policy used by armies which treat first of all those soldiers most likely to return quickly to the battle.

7 To make apparently reflective judgements merely a matter of calculation.

Against QALYs

Before considering further objections to the use of QALYs it is important to place the current controversy in a more general perspective. The debate actually represents nothing more than the swing of a pendulum between deontology and consequentialism. At present there is great emphasis on the assessment of the consequences of actions, as a gauge to their worth. But this fashion – and it is nothing more – misses so much of importance in human life, and misses it so blatantly, that it will not last for long: cutting costs is a pointless exercise if it is done only for its own sake. (Indeed, in 2008, there is less talk about consequences and much more talk about 'putting the patient first', 'service user involvement' and 'basing health services on clear statements of value'.[97])

Sooner or later any form of utilitarianism becomes absurd if it is not part of a wider picture. For example, Jeremy Bentham invented the Felicific Calculus,[98] meant to help people decide what to do, based on an assessment of likely consequences (roughly, the more pleasure an action is likely to produce the more reason to do it). Bentham took into account the type, intensity and duration of pleasure, and argued for a standard scale by which to calculate. His hope was that everyone would agree on this standard. But, just like QALYs, his strategy was doomed to failure because different people have different ideas about how to rate pleasures. Imagine, for illustration, how difficult it would be for any group of people from dissimilar backgrounds to agree about the relative merits of reading a good novel, eating a large bar of chocolate, getting drunk with friends on Saturday night, robbing a bank or whatever other entertainment is proposed.

In defence of the Felicific Calculus it should be said that Bentham took other people's pleasures into account, arguing that the worth of human actions should be seen against a background of pleasure generated overall. However, just as they share inability to settle on objective measures, in application both Bentham's Calculus and QALYs flounder ethically, because they can legitimise extravagant discrimination. So long as the general balance is more 'good' than 'bad' then actions – whatever they are – are said to be justified (for Bentham the 'good' is pleasure and the 'bad' pain, while for the advocates of QALYs, life protected cheaply is 'good' while expensive life is 'bad').

Both ways of calculation are deeply contrary to justice as fairness. It is worth recalling an illustration to emphasise the point. If we are given the option of having a disease-free, war-free, content and wholly productive society at the single cost of knowing that one human being will be kept in eternal and perpetual agony of mind and body, should we accept? If they are honest, consequentialists (and therefore almost all economists) have to agree to the contract – or else relinquish all consistency – yet the injustice of the situation is obvious.

The following specific points may be made against QALYs.

1 Their content is arbitrary

QALY criteria – degree of pain, length of expected life and degree of disability – are at worst arbitrary and at best governed by a health service preoccupied with economics, mortality and morbidity. In the absence of a theory of health service purpose, there is no reason why these components should have been chosen before, for example, intelligence, amount of past income, amount of body hair, height or eye colour. Why not these measures? If a person was unfortunate enough to be completely bald, quite small, rather stupid and to have been unemployed for a long time it might be concluded that her quality of life is low, and that someone else ought to be treated in her stead.

These criteria would quickly be condemned as unfair and arbitrary – discriminating solely according to a person's bad luck – but of course this is precisely what the QALY measure does. The criteria might sound more objective, gaining credibility from the traditional medical context, but they have been selected from an indefinite range of alternatives. If you are old or disabled or in pain or immobile – tough luck. It does not matter that you devote your life to charity – you are 78 and not worth as much as the 25-year-old businessman with two children.

2 QALYs impose subjective values on other subjects (and claim objectivity as they do so)[94]

Their use to discriminate between people means that arbitrary or biased criteria are imposed on those who do not share their way of thinking. Worse still, many economists[99] claim their advice is unbiased, or value-neutral, when this is patently not the case.

3 QALYs promote many myths

Among them:

a. That it is possible to be certain about the outcomes of treatment, that we know how long people will live, that my pain is the same as your pain, and that the QALY calculation can be carried out without difficulty and without assumptions.

b. That in all cases where QALYs are used to discriminate it is feasible to calculate what to do. The idea that each human being is unique, and that each of us has defining qualities that cannot be measured, is not considered. Just as only a partial aspect of moral reasoning is recognised, it is assumed that all health services cases are, by and large, governed by the same few factors.[62]

The selection of 'easy' cases as examples helps further this latter myth. For instance, if the choice lies between offering scarce life-saving treatment to a 35-year-old man with a good career and a young family, or to help a 70-year-old with no close relatives then – all else being equal – QALYs explain why it makes sense to discriminate against the older man. But it is a different matter if the choice is between a 13-year-old boy and an 11-year-old girl. If only one can be treated and the primary discriminatory measure – length of expected life and treatment cost – are not applicable, and all other selected criteria are equal, then the QALY is no help at all. The reason why it is morally difficult to discriminate between two children is that we have a deep feeling they are entitled to equal respect and so equal treatment. And the feeling remains in the case of the 35-year-old and the 70-year-old – why are these two people not entitled to equal respect if the boy and girl are?

4 The slippery slope

It should by now be obvious how easily the acceptance of QALYs makes it to slide down a slope where injustice to some can be 'justified' as being in the interest of the majority. This is the justification Hitler used to explain the murder of Jews – it was said to be in the interest of the German nation as a whole – and the justification of apartheid.

QALYs inevitably discriminate on the ground of age, and can readily be used to discriminate on grounds of race, sex or class. If you are old then your life expectancy is usually less than if you are young, so if there is to be a straight choice between the old and the young the old must be sacrificed, regardless of how much they want to live, how much they have to give, or how much they value their futures.

If you are a woman your life expectancy is longer than a man's, therefore you should receive the scarce resource – all other things being equal. But if you are a woman you might suffer from some medical conditions men do not. If the treatment for these is more expensive than the treatment for his, and there is not enough money to go round, then you might find that you will not be treated yet he will.

Epidemiological studies inform us that different races suffer from different diseases and have different life expectancies. So do the different classes. A member of parliament can expect a longer life then a mineworker, so again – all other things being equal – the MP should be treated at the expense of the mineworker.

It does not require a massive leap of imagination to understand how QALYs could be used to justify non-voluntary euthanasia, or allowing handicapped infants to die, or the abandonment of mental patients of no danger to society. Defenders of QALYs might argue that safeguards could be built into the system, and already exist in most Western legislation, but if that is so reassuring why not pick a better system in the first place?

The benefit of QALYs

The main benefit of open discussion about QALYs is that they expose the implicit, though often unintentional and unavoidable, injustice of some decisions taken in the present health service – injustice that might be avoided given different structure and funding. QALYs remind us that health service resources are usually scarce, not as a result of nature but as a consequence of a human decision to spend money elsewhere, for instance on weapons of war, on luxuries, on fast cars, on houses with more rooms than we need and so on. Spending on weapons, for instance, is usually 'justified' on the ground that they act to preserve human life by deterring warmongers. But the preservation of human life is a central role for medical services too, and in a more direct and continuous sense. Since war is not imminent there is surely a case (which bad faith tends to obscure) that at least some military defence money be transferred to medical services constantly involved in the defence of human life.

What should be done?

John Harris has proposed that the only fair way to distribute a scarce resource is to draw lots. If, for instance, there are 10 potential patients and only one bed available in an intensive care unit then clinical circumstances should not be taken into account; rather the decision should be left to chance. The patient who draws the longest straw should be helped – even if she stands less chance of a good recovery than her fellow gamblers. This is fair in the sense that everyone has an equal chance, but is it practicable? Would any doctor ever carry out such a lottery? It seems unlikely, not least because the doctor would almost certainly face legal action if she did.

We are now left with two unacceptable alternatives: to discriminate between people as a matter of policy – thus offending a basic principle of civilised society that all people are entitled to equal respect, regardless of their luck or their talents – or to be undiscriminating, drawing lots for a scant resources. But this seems neither practical nor cost-effective. Randomness by itself does not amount to a policy of equal respect. How could a doctor explain to a mother that her young child had been sacrificed as the result of a lottery, to save an old man with only months left to live?

What is needed is experience, consideration and the ability to reason morally

Sometimes hard choices have to be faced. Where decisions have to be made about who to treat and who not to treat doctors need guidance. It is not entirely immoral to treat the 15-year-old rather than the 95-year-old, or the 25-year-old with a minor illness rather than the terminally ill 25-year-old, but in order to show this a complete deliberation is necessary – not just an economic one.

Because each situation is unique the idea of applying a crude quantitative measure only is unsuitable. What is worse, the use of QALYs might turn doctors into calculating machines where they come to believe that moral judgements are a matter of measuring simple differences. Once this has become habit doctors might begin to think that computed answers are not their responsibility but somehow objective, disregarding the fact they have chosen to use the measure in the first place. What is needed is not an unjust technique but responsible, caring individuals and organisations – humane systems, not purely economic ones.

Four practical proposals:

1 That education in moral reasoning be given to all medical practitioners and health workers, on a regular basis. Health workers should be given education in analysis of interventions, in weighing up strengths and weaknesses of alternatives, in the use of logic, in law, and in the assessment of duties and consequences.

It should be explained that ethics is a process of deliberation in which it is necessary to select certain priorities from a range of possibilities. In any ethical deliberation in health work four levels should be addressed: external considerations such as evidence for one's judgement, duties, consequences and the core rationale of health work. Once this core is understood health workers will know that the unqualified use of QALYs is not proper work for health.

2 In particular, every health authority should use a Values Exchange (www.values-exchange.com), and all employees should be required to complete one reflective analysis per month.
3 Every health authority should include as many service users as possible in Values Exchange (www.values-exchange.com) deliberations – so that the professionals can clearly include service users' perspectives in their decision-making, and so that service users can more clearly understand the decision-making pressures the professionals are under.
4 That since 'scarce resources' are scarce only as a result of lack of funds which might be available from other sources, and since by the use of statistics it is possible to predict fairly accurately how many dialysis machines and other such resources will be needed, it should become public knowledge that lives are being lost and those doctors who must decide are being placed in impossible positions as a result of human priorities, not natural circumstances.

Consequently, whenever a health worker has to make a 'tragic choice' – sacrificing a life where that life could have been saved – there should be a recognised professional facility for this to be publicly recorded. This could be done through medical associations, who could ensure accuracy, and publicised each month in national newspapers. Since newspapers regularly print stories of murder and road death as examples of avoidable injustice this should not be unappealing to them.

It might even be desirable to have a league table of 'enforced injustice in medicine'.

Conclusions

This chapter has outlined obstacles in the path of clear moral reasoning. Such obstacles should be avoided by health workers. If they are not overcome it will not be possible to use the Ethical Grid or the Values Exchange (www.values-exchange.com).

The Rings of Uncertainty

Introduction

The penultimate parts of this book offer two decision-support devices to health workers: the Rings of Uncertainty (this chapter) and the Ethical Grid (**Chapter Nine**). Both were originally designed as paper-based prompts to personal and small group reflection. They were meant to stimulate thought in readers and groups by suggesting multiple perspectives on situations, and by providing simple to understand frameworks on which to hang and organise those thoughts.

Both the Rings of Uncertainty and the Ethical Grid have become part of the Values Exchange (www.values-exchange.com), and have evolved further in the process. Their use in the Values Exchange (www.values-exchange.com) is explained in **Chapter Twelve**. Readers may be interested to compare their original incarnation (explained in the next two chapters) with what they have now become (which can be seen by registering here, for example: www.staffs.values-exchange.co.uk/register).

This chapter suggests a way for health workers to picture their positions in a world of uncertainty. By means of this they will be better placed to judge the most desirable courses to steer.

'What role ought a health worker adopt?' 'What should limit her activity?' At the moment health workers are guided primarily by precedent and vague subjective judgement. Apart from the Ethical Grid there is no substantial framework to help a health worker arrive at a systematically reasoned position. As a result it is often difficult for other health workers – doctors, nurses, managers and patients – to challenge the reasoning processes that led to an intervention. The vague phrase 'I exercised my clinical/nursing/managerial judgement' is still used to conceal woolly or dubious thinking – and other health professionals do not possess a mutual structure to enable encouragement or restraint. If a nurse thinks a doctor is not doing enough to help a patient, or a manager believes a nurse is going too far, there is no shared logical means by which to facilitate discussion. Consequently, confrontation regularly occurs where constructive conversation might have been.

By presenting a graphic, graspable model for health workers to reflect upon possible roles and interventions, this chapter attempts to increase understanding of the philosophical basis of health work. It also suggests a means of enhancing communication between health workers of all kinds – to the benefit of those for whom they care.

The Rings of Uncertainty

The Rings can best be explained in a series of steps.

Step One

Represented generally in Figure 29, uncertainty is the most abiding and pervasive limit on health work.

The traditional aim of health work is to move from the outside to the inside – to come ever closer to certainty. However, when this abstract idea is specifically expressed it can be seen that inward progress is not necessarily the most appropriate direction. For instance, it is sometimes better that a doctor moves outwards in the Rings – especially if she thinks of herself as a general problem-solver who wants to work for health. Although this may not be the safest option – it becomes more likely she will be exposed to criticism, for instance – there are considerable benefits to be had. For example, by stretching outwards a doctor might learn from other people and so extend her competence, she might discover fresh and broader options for problem-solving, new approaches and methods might become apparent and – perhaps most important of all – by welcoming

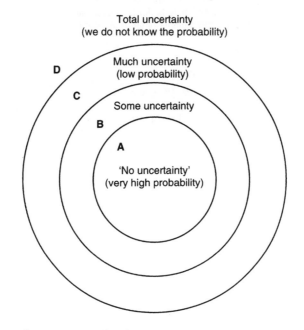

Figure 29 The Rings of Uncertainty in the abstract

the idea of outward travel rather than constantly seeking shelter in certainty, her flexibility may increase. She may learn when to be humble and when it is best to be passive. Indeed it is only by facing outwards as well as inwards that anyone can work for health in the richest sense.[100]

The basic diagram can be adapted to show each limit to health work. Consider first the Rings expressed for technical competence.

Step Two: the Rings expressed

Technical competence

Technical competence includes both knowledge and skill. Competence (or lack of it) comes in many guises. Figure 30 translates the idea into a form suitable for the Rings of Uncertainty.

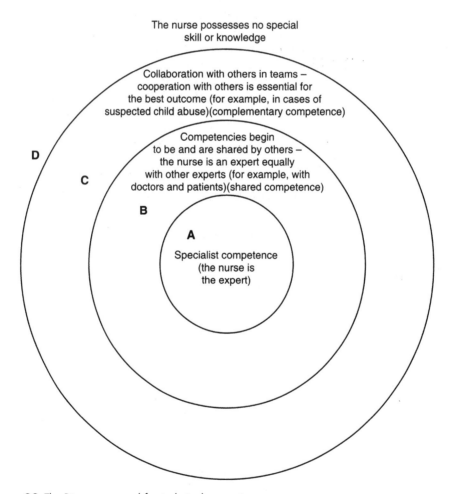

The nurse possesses no special skill or knowledge

Collaboration with others in teams – cooperation with others is essential for the best outcome (for example, in cases of suspected child abuse)(complementary competence)

Competencies begin to be and are shared by others – the nurse is an expert equally with other experts (for example, with doctors and patients)(shared competence)

D

C

B

A

Specialist competence (the nurse is the expert)

Figure 30 The Rings expressed for technical competence

As with any general framework, the words used to describe each Ring can mean different things in different circumstances. For instance, the competencies in question might be competencies of technique, insight or recall of information. When the Rings are expressed for resources these might be human organs, money, beds, time or skilled people – whatever might legitimately be considered a resource. Reality must give meaning to each Ring.

Figure 30 is a simple representation of one way in which nursing activity might be limited by competence. It is better not to imagine a nurse jumping from one section of the Rings to another. Although the Rings as illustrated appear sharply divided, in reality different levels of competence shade into each other, just as a bold scarlet can fade slowly to the palest pink. The Rings are meant to convey a steady weakening of certainty as the nurse moves towards the outer edge.

Different sorts of question are likely to arise dependent upon the nurse's perceived position. For example, is the nurse the only person in a position to offer help? Should she intervene only with the advice and assistance of others? Is the nurse's ability to help so limited that any intervention is ill-advised?

Imagine how Sally Smith might use the Rings. Sally is a nurse who has established a relationship with John Jones, a cancer patient who also suffers from moderate depression. Sally has used the Rings before and is able to picture herself actually and potentially within them. She knows that by thinking graphically she is sometimes able to reason more concretely. By using the Rings Sally can say 'if I do that, then I shall be standing in this position within the Rings of Uncertainty'. In one sense this is to do no more than say 'if I do this, X will happen', but Sally has discovered that reference to the image can deepen her thought processes.

John – a bachelor of 31 – has cancer of the bone. His doctors advise that an operation now would give him a 50% chance of a cure, but they will have to amputate his arm below the left elbow. John was distraught to learn this. To lose a limb has always been one of his biggest dreads, and to make matters worse he makes his living playing the guitar.

John refused to consent to the operation and was told that any other treatment is probably useless. In shock he informs Sally that he wishes to discharge himself from hospital.

Sally has an ethical problem to deal with, of course. However, in order to decide what to do she needs more than ethical theory. She really needs to work out *where she stands* in this situation, and thinks the Rings might help.

She considers the Rings expressed for competence, as shown in Figure 30. Where does she see herself? She is in the outer rings for medical knowledge, though she is by no means a novice in oncology. But she does not have *special* knowledge, and to do anything clinical for John she would clearly have to work with a team. However, she has specialised in counselling and communication, and is the most qualified person in the department in this respect. She also knows John better than anyone else – she is a similar age and they have had several chats over the last couple of days.

If she had been a poor communicator – and had pictured herself standing at the edges of the Rings expressed for competence in this regard – she would probably have been best advised to let John leave, or to refer him on. However, not only is she in the centre ring but the doctors have little interest in John now – they think he has made a bad decision but they cannot and will not do anything without his consent – and they have compliant patients to assist.

She resolves to set time aside to talk with John, to help him think his decision through. He agrees to this, and says he will wait in hospital until the end of her shift. As she talks with him he tells her he cannot live as a freak and cannot imagine how he will survive without his music. Sally calmly puts an opposite view and – with John's permission – introduces him to two amputees, who visit people like John. They too are in the middle of this set of Rings in these circumstances.

Unfortunately, Sally's strategy does not have the hoped for effect. John breaks down in extreme distress. He cries and begins to rage loudly against his ill-fortune – he accuses the medics of maltreating him. At this Sally realises she is no longer in the middle ring. At best she is at B, in a situation where other people are equally as expert as she, and she may well be at C. Knowing this she holds John, and manages to comfort and soothe him. He says he will wait on the ward while she goes to see what can be done.

Sally calls a psychiatrist and another nurse counsellor from elsewhere in the hospital. She returns to John, who agrees to see them – and the situation moves on. If it is to be resolved it will require multi-disciplinary effort and clear ethical reasoning – in fact it is now time for Sally, her colleagues and John to employ the Ethical Grid. Yet the Rings have been crucial in the early stages – without them Sally might not have felt it appropriate to intervene without the permission of her clinical colleagues, and there would now be less chance of helping John deal with his crisis.

Other expressions of the Rings

The general Rings (Figure 29 – stretching from a core where confidence can be at a peak to a surrounding area where there is no ground for professional intervention) can be translated into several other categories. Health workers are free to suggest their own if they find the Rings helpful, or they may prefer to choose from the following selection.

Resources

Broader picturing: resources plus technical competence
The following brief example (Figure 31) shows how complexity can begin to deepen. Envisage Dr Smith, a consultant surgeon, standing within the Rings of Uncertainty expressed for resources. In order to work to greatest effect, to direct his time and energy along the most profitable channels, he must understand his position accurately within the Rings expressed in this way. Where he can stand will depend on the extent of the resources available, and might also change according to his interpretation of the word 'resource'.

In order to arrive at the best practical approach Dr Smith should try to see himself standing simultaneously within other expressions of the Rings of Uncertainty: as if two or more Rings were superimposed one on another. For instance, if he would like to perform a heart transplant it is certain there will be resource issues. But inevitably there will be other variables to consider, of which technical competence will be one.

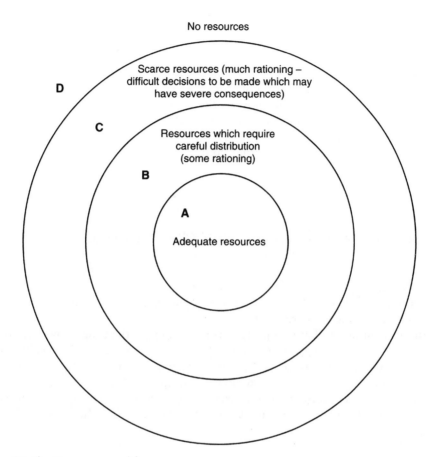

No resources

Scarce resources (much rationing –
difficult decisions to be made which may
have severe consequences)

D

C

Resources which require
careful distribution
(some rationing)

B

A

Adequate resources

Figure 31 The Rings expressed for resources

As far as resources are concerned, if a suitable donor organ cannot be obtained Dr Smith will be stranded in the area surrounding the Rings (D). If a compatible heart does become available then the doctor will either be operating within the outer circle (C) (where the heart is a scarce resource, and where he may have to decide who will be given it) or, if there is only one patient awaiting an organ, he will be operating within the centre ring (A), with adequate resources in this sense at least. In this respect Dr Smith's position within the Rings is entirely subject to prevailing circumstances.

Perhaps Dr Smith wishes to transplant a kidney, has an adequate supply in his locality, but does not have sufficient funding from his health authority or hospital to pay for support staff to provide a full service. And as a consequence patients are suffering, and in some cases dying, where they need not. In this case then he is actually standing in either (C) (much rationing) or (B) (some rationing) rings, but will almost certainly be seeking to stand within the centre ring (A) (adequate resources).

If he wishes to make progress – if he wishes to be creative with the various limits in which he finds himself – then Dr Smith may have to consider the extent of his role within limits other than resources. For instance, if he wishes to change the situation he may have to ponder where he stands within the Rings expressed for competence, and work out where he might move within these Rings.

At present he is a single consultant lacking staff. With the advantage of his professional status he can put some pressure on hospital management, but cannot be confident he will win his way. He may have to move out from the centre to the second or third rings – perhaps to the third ring – where he must work in a team with other consultants, or with other health workers. If he really wants to do something in these circumstances then Dr Smith must imagine himself standing within two sets of Rings at once, and must consider where he should stand for the best within both.

Law

Health care is a complex and uncertain affair. Given this, and given that change to a simpler system is not foreseeable, the prudent health worker will seek to recognise his position in the Rings expressed for law (Figure 32) – for he may wish to alter his practice dependent upon his perceived position. For example, he may choose to practise 'defensive medicine/nursing',[101] and so be ultra-cautious whenever he pictures himself in the third ring (C), where the law is unpredictable.

The effect picturing can have on practice is not unique to the Rings expressed for law. For instance, when the Rings are expressed for technical competence a health worker may decide to be decisively in charge (perhaps when a patient sincerely asks him to do so, when a patient is very ill or unconscious, or deeply frightened) or clearly an agent for his patient, respecting the patient's beliefs and choices entirely. The health worker need not always do what a patient wants – though he must always seek to create autonomy.

Within the Rings expressed for law

How should a nurse conceive of herself and her activity? And how might such picturing affect her actions? How might this help define a limit around what she might do?

Consider Emma Halsall, a practice nurse encouraged by her health centre to carry out simple surgical techniques, rather than refer patients on for more expensive treatment. Where should she place himself within the Rings expressed for law when a patient asks her to remove a verruca from her foot?

Should Emma picture herself in the centre ring (A) (where the law is clear) or in another? If she thinks of herself as standing in the centre, by implication she believes she need worry only about gaining the patient's consent for the operation, so as not to risk an accusation of battery. Given this, so long as she lives up to the standard set by the Bolam Test[102] (if she is in England and Wales) she need not reflect further – particularly if she also sees herself standing within the centre of the Rings expressed for technical competence and communication. But would Emma not be wise at least to picture herself within the second ring (B), where she chances some danger of litigation if things go wrong? If she does so she might then take great care that the operated area does not become infected, perhaps to the extent that she asks the patient back daily to check the

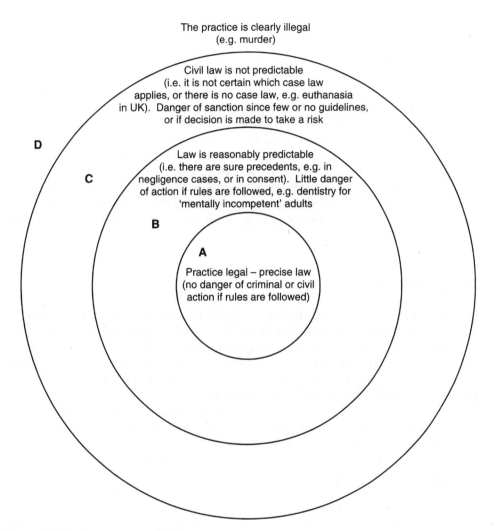

The practice is clearly illegal
(e.g. murder)

Civil law is not predictable
(i.e. it is not certain which case law
applies, or there is no case law, e.g. euthanasia
in UK). Danger of sanction since few or no guidelines,
or if decision is made to take a risk

Law is reasonably predictable
(i.e. there are sure precedents, e.g. in
negligence cases, or in consent). Little danger
of action if rules are followed, e.g. dentistry for
'mentally incompetent' adults

Practice legal – precise law
(no danger of criminal or civil
action if rules are followed)

D

C

B

A

Figure 32 The Rings expressed for law

wound. Of course, in order to decide this question, she will need to picture herself within Rings expressed for other contents, particularly technical competence and resources.

Tension between different Rings
Since the Rings merely reflect considerations that must be taken into account in real-life decision-making it is often the case that, although a health worker may wish to place himself at certain points within Rings expressed for different contents, he will not be able to stand where he wants simultaneously in each Ring. Health workers can wish to move in different directions at once, and there can be irreconcilable tensions between desired positions within the Rings in some situations.

Take the case of Dr Greaves, who is consulted by a 57-year-old, retired, heavy smoking, 4 st overweight bus-driver with a history of angina, who says that he has had to stop and sit down for 15 minutes whilst walking because he was so short of breath, and felt some pain in his chest. Should Dr Greaves decide to sit plumb in the centre of the Rings expressed for law and examine the man thoroughly, before referring him to the appropriate hospital consultant – or to A&E – in order to attempt to prevent a possible heart attack? If he does this then he will be extremely prudent, but he will also use up valuable time. Alternatively, should Dr Greaves place himself at the centre of the Rings expressed for resources, taking care to ensure he has adequate time for each of his patients, whilst accepting the risk involved with a move into the third ring (C) of the Rings expressed for law? If he decides to stand in (C) ring, if he decides to send the bus-driver away after a cursory examination, then he will have placed himself in danger of an accusation of negligence – of not meeting the accepted standard of care of the competent general practitioner. What if the bus-driver actually suffers a heart attack?

Communication

The breadth of existing language, both general and technical, will inescapably limit the extent of communication between health workers, and between health workers and patients. The study of language and communication is a complex subject.[103] The aspect of most concern to health professionals is usually the extent to which meaning is understood: does the patient/client have a clear picture of what I have said? Have I properly grasped what the patient is trying to describe to me?

Consider pain. Pain can be an intensely meaningful word, but is notoriously difficult to translate accurately. When a person is asked if she feels pain she is commonly asked for its location and severity, and most of us can relate this. But if more detail is needed it is difficult, if not impossible, to tell whether intended meaning has been correctly conveyed. If she explains that the pain is 'stabbing' or 'deep' or 'intense' this may not be enough to establish a clear clinical picture without further investigation. And even if it is sufficient for a clinical assessment, it may nonetheless not put across a faithful representation of the pain. If a more detailed and extensive 'pain language' could be devised and made common currency then the limits of language might stretch to allow more extensive communication.

There are other examples of the way the limit on what may be communicated can expand. For instance, the language of psychiatry develops regularly.[104] And as new technology is invented (for example, 'body scanning' by 'magnetic resonance' or 'genetic engineering') so new words and uses of language become necessary to describe the images produced. Equally, the limits may shrink.

Some commentators[105] have argued that this process occurred in the 1960s when 'reductionist science' enjoyed its heyday. (Reductionism is the belief that the way to understand more about nature is to gain knowledge about ever smaller parts of it. Thus it might be held that more can be learnt about disease through biochemistry than through social research.)

During this era words and phrases such as 'holistic', 'spiritual healing' and 'person-centred' were considered empty by many scientists.

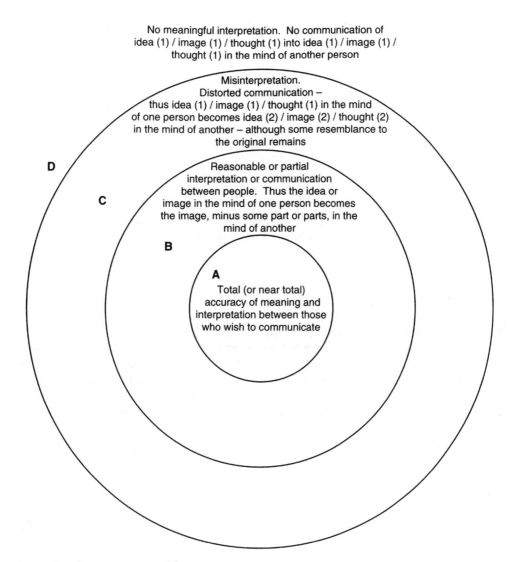

Figure 33 The Rings expressed for communication

Figure 33 suggests one way of representing levels of communication using the Rings of Uncertainty. The wording implies language in the sense of shared meaning between those who wish to communicate.

This is only one possible formulation of the Rings expressed for language and communication. The simple model cannot, without over-stretching credibility and coherence, accommodate all possibilities. It is one simple model of communication among the many that can be found in work in the philosophy of language. No attempt is made here to deal with its philosophical difficulties – for instance, how does one actually check whether idea (1) remains idea (1) or has become idea (3)? However, it will suffice for the most familiar difficulties of language use. It is not uncommon to underestimate the extent of these, and the levels of language and communication are therefore an important inclusion.

For example, whether using technical or common language, it is often not clear that full comprehension has occurred. It is well known that the use of technical terms without explanation can generate confusion. As we have seen, 'ethics' has a variety of meanings. For some 'ethics' means 'a personal code of behaviour' and for others 'rules governing society'. And while 'therapy' may be a neutral or enabling activity for most therapists, for some patients the word can carry connotations of blame and punishment. Some patients assume they are responsible for their illness, and see therapy as a form of penance – 'I would not need therapy had I been a better person'. If what is meant is not specified clearly then misunderstanding is likely.

Misunderstandings can occur as the result of under-elaboration (for example, 'go to bed and take bed-rest' might imply a day or a week of confinement); misperception of emphasis (for example, 'this operation has some risk, like all operations' might mean one thing to the doctor and quite another to the patient, not least because it is the patient who must undergo the operation and the doctor who must perform or observe it); and misinterpretation through ambiguity (for example, the words 'safe', 'cancer' and 'love' have a range of meanings). A good health worker must be careful that comprehension is as accurate as possible. It can be a valuable exercise for a health worker habitually to attempt to picture herself within the Rings expressed this way.

Although the Rings are not intended for urgent situations it can be helpful to have them in mind during some consultations. In especially fraught meetings the level of understanding can quickly change. Some news can have a dramatic effect on communication. To take one example, in a discussion between a doctor and patient from similar backgrounds (both professionals, both white, both men, both middle-class and both in their fifties) about the results of exploratory tests, communication may take place within either Rings (A) or (B), until a certain point in the conversation. Having explained the background to the tests, and having imparted some key factual information about the test process, when the doctor announces 'I'm afraid the results show that you have an advanced malignancy – I'm sorry Jeff, you have cancer', the consultation leaps to levels (C) or (D). Both the doctor and patient now inhabit an area of heightened uncertainty.

While a person is shocked any communication is likely to be less meaningful. The Rings can be a reminder of the need to adapt one's work to a new set of circumstances. In addition, the fact that the level of communication has changed may affect the position of the doctor or health worker within the Rings expressed in other ways. For example, movement may be necessary within Rings expressed for resources, since more time may be required. Similarly, because shock can adversely affect the reasoning process, a fresh positioning within the Rings expressed for law and ethics might be necessary if a question of informed consent arises. If there is a serious problem of communication it may be that the Rings expressed in these ways assume the highest significance – if only temporarily.

It is now possible for a health worker who wishes to gain a clearer insight into the limits of his role to picture himself standing within the Rings of Uncertainty expressed for competence, resources, law and communication. Intriguingly, he might see himself standing at a different level for each expression of the Rings, and might notice pulls and tensions if his imagination runs contrary to reality.

But although the Rings are potentially illuminating, the model is getting confused. Simplification and more exact guidance is required. However, before this notice that a crucial difference becomes apparent when the Rings are expressed for ethics. Whereas it is possible to offer acceptable, albeit simplistic, terminology to express the Rings in other ways, it is difficult if not impossible for ethics.

Ethics

Two immediate difficulties are encountered when attempting to express the Rings for ethics (Figure 34). First, the labels appear so open to interpretation they seem to cover many different interventions. Second, where one person chooses to imagine himself standing may not be the place another person would put him for the same intervention. And there seems no definite way to resolve such a disagreement.

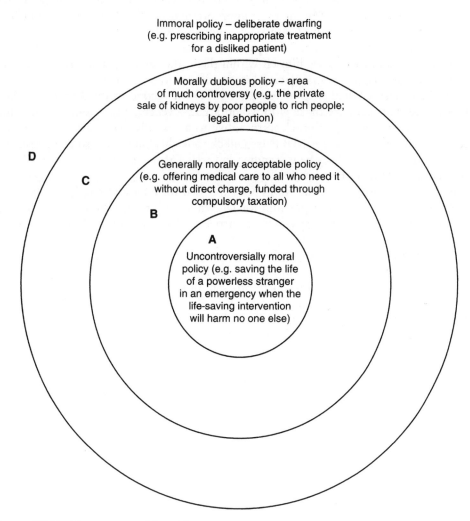

Figure 34 The Rings expressed for ethics

Consider Dr White, a general practitioner, who is wondering what advice (or device) to offer Joanne who has come to see him with a request for a prescription for the contraceptive pill.

Joanne is just 15. She is categorised by those who find such classification useful as lower working class, and has a strong accent and use of English peculiar to her locality. Dr White sees he has an ethical problem. He also appreciates that he could usefully visualise himself as standing within the Rings of Uncertainty translated in other ways. For example, he might choose to express them for language and communication. Alternatively he might choose to express the Rings for law – focusing on the legal controversy that surrounded the Gillick case in the 1980s.[106,107] However, Dr White decides that on balance his best option is to imagine himself standing within the Rings expressed for ethics.

The doctor has not been confronted with a case like this before, but is inclined towards any policy that helps other people and respects their wishes. Consequently, as Joanne begins to blurt out she wants the Pill, his basic instinct is to talk it through with her and then, all being well, to prescribe the most appropriate drug. Dr White decides to clarify his position – because he knows his instinct is not shared by all doctors, and suspects it might be important to analyse his position. But, as he conjures up his mental picture of a series of rings and tries to see himself within them, the image is muddled. He can see himself (and can imagine others placing him) within more than one circle.

Dr White is unsure whether to imagine himself in the second or third rings, and he is further aware that there are those who would argue – vehemently in some cases – that by considering prescribing an oral contraceptive to a sexually active girl under the age of consent he is standing in area (D) (Mrs Gillick took this line). He also recognises that there are some who would say he is standing in Circle (A) (people in the Women's Rights Movement usually take this view).

There is a peculiarity when the Rings are expressed for ethics: it is unlikely there will be consensus about the correct position for Dr White within the ethics Rings, yet if the Rings are expressed for law or resources controversy does not persist. In these cases Dr White's position will be open to empirical verification. The current law is that doctors can prescribe the pill to under-age girls of sufficient maturity, though they must make efforts to encourage each girl to inform her parents or guardians.[108] And there are adequate supplies of the Pill, so no resource problem in this case.

As we have seen throughout this book, ethics always involves value judgements and is therefore not easy to represent in the Rings image. Ethics pervades health work, so an accurate representation would somehow show ethics saturating the Rings – since health work is a moral endeavour any application of the Rings requires ethical reflection. However, for practical reasons it is better to show ethics as a segment of the analytic process. So long as the reasoner knows this the Rings can be used to good pragmatic effect. (Note: the above paragraphs strongly anticipated the Values Exchange: www.values-exchange.com.)

The limits of health work – from insight to guidance

It is too much to expect a health worker to retain five (or possibly more) Rings in her mind, and then to judge accurately what her role ought to be. The model needs further development.

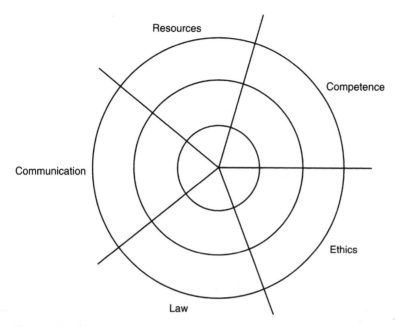

Resources

Competence

Communication

Ethics

Law

Figure 35 The various expressions united

Step Three

It is possible to simplify the Rings of Uncertainty by making use of only one set of Rings divided into various segments (Figure 35).

Step Four

Making use of the single set of Rings, it is suggested that during the process of conceiving – during the process of picturing his position – a health worker experiments, placing markers in what he considers the appropriate sections of the segmented rings. He may decide he does not require every segment during this process. It may be that for a particular problem, a health worker thinks the main considerations are resources, competence, law and ethics, and so chooses to divide the Rings as illustrated (Figure 36).

Perhaps the doctor is a general practitioner who has to decide whether to perform a minor operation. On thinking about it, using one segmented Ring with markers, he may come up with an image like Figure 37.

This image depicts the doctor's decision. In order to arrive at it, the doctor had to consider each category. He decided he has adequate resources – he has the correct equipment, time and staff support. But where technical competence is concerned he must collaborate with others – he needs detailed advice from a consultant surgeon colleague. Ethically he thinks the policy is dubious. He worries it is a potentially risky form of

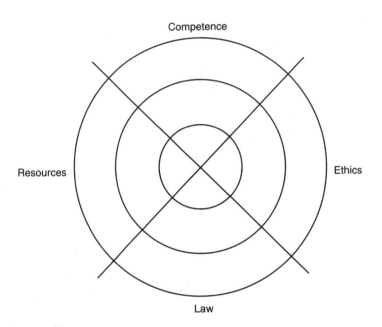

Figure 36 One possible set-up

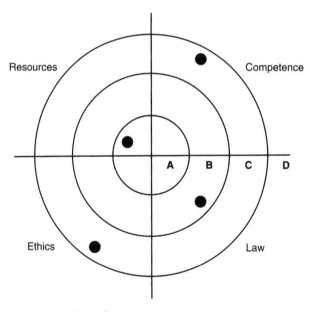

Figure 37 A segmented Ring with markers

cost-cutting, and that a better result might be achieved in a hospital. He also fears litigation, primarily because of his position within the technical competence segment.

On balance the GP decides not to do it. But his decision was imprecise. It would be
possible, but very cumbersome, to translate the decision-making process into a series of
hypotheses and tests. A doctor might begin by forming the hypothesis, *if I operate in my*

surgery, I run no extraordinary risk. He might then express the possible risks in terms of the categories he has selected, and assess these separately, perhaps arriving at different conclusions for law and ethics. At a later point he might test the hypothesis, *by seeking the advice of a specialist surgeon, I minimise the risk of litigation if the operation is not a success*. But this would be only one among many hypotheses he would need to test.

Naturally such exhaustive hypothesis generation and testing is rarely if ever undertaken in the clinical context. Judging and reasoning is a more fluid and agile human process than this. Fortunately, however, it is possible to add further precision to the Rings.

Step Five

A key dictum

It should be obvious to all health workers that if introspection shows them standing outside the Rings of Uncertainty they ought not intervene. This is a clear practical limit to health work. If the potential intervention appears immoral, illegal and beyond communication, and the worker has no resources and is incompetent, then only a fool would do it. Indeed, if the health worker thinks she is outside the Rings for any segment it is doubtful she should act.

It is possible to derive a key dictum from this that *if a health worker's imagination shows him standing outside the Rings for any segment then this is a very strong indication that a limit to health work has been reached*. Unless the circumstances are exceptional, the worker should not proceed.

However, there may be exceptional circumstances. It may be that for some segments at least, to stand beyond the Rings will not necessarily require the abandonment of the project. For instance, just because an action is illegal it is not always out of the question, especially if the doctor is simultaneously standing within the Rings expressed for ethics. In some people's eyes euthanasia is a perfect example of this.

As a general guide it can be said that the further towards the edges of the Rings a health worker sees herself standing, the more reason she has to question the wisdom of her situation or plan. But this guideline is still too general to be of much practical use. What if the health worker has divided her Rings of Uncertainty into four segments and conceives of herself as standing in the centre for two and at the edges of the outer ring for the other two segments? How is she to assess her most appropriate role in these circumstances?

One option, of course, is to use the Ethical Grid to assist a process of detailed moral reasoning (so overriding the Rings). She might make this move straight away, if she wishes, but it is still possible to discover more precision using only the Rings.

Step Six

The Rings cannot be used abstractly. Dependent upon content and circumstance the importance of any segment will vary. Noting this, further life can be breathed into the Rings by granting movement to the segments, to allow their area to fluctuate in size.

The lines dividing the segments can now pivot around the centre-point of the Rings, and can be altered like the hands on a carriage-clock.

Thus it may be that if a nurse manager decides, for a particular case, that there are three key considerations (say, technical competence, resources and law) she will not be restricted to a static model of this type (Figure 38).

Instead she will be able to reflect upon her decision by according each consideration a relative importance (Figure 39).

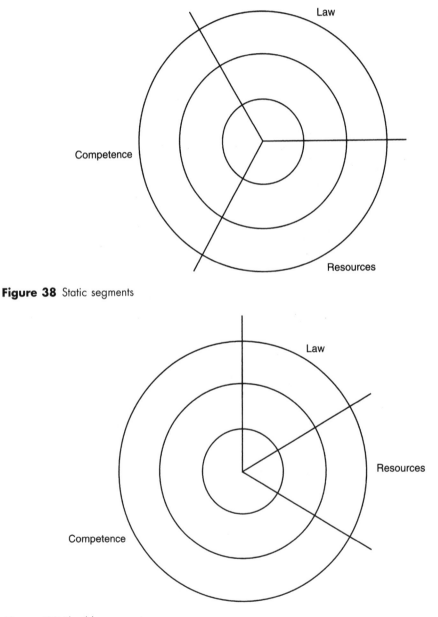

Figure 38 Static segments

Figure 39 Flexible segments

By altering the segments in such a way the manager indicates that her skill and knowledge are the main concern in this case. Her decision about where she stands within the Rings expressed for competence will have a crucial influence on the decision taken.

Scoring and quantification

The Rings of Uncertainty are designed primarily as conceptual guidelines, not to provide rigid, quantifiable rulings. However, it might be that individual health workers will wish to invent a personal scoring system, particularly if their specialisation is such that they tend to conceive most or all of their markers placed neither in the centre nor on the outside of the Rings whenever they have to make a decision. It may be that for some a system of numbers could prove decisive in borderline cases, where a doctor (for instance) must choose whether or not to go ahead with an intervention. As one means of orientation a doctor might decide to score the centre of the Rings as 4, the next ring as 3, the outer ring as 2, and the surrounding area as 0. She might decide she will add up the scores for each ring, divide by the number of segments, and accept a cut-off point of say, less than 3, as a guide that she should not proceed. If she chooses a lower cut-off point, then she will be choosing to take greater risks, but may find other benefits along the way.

To act as a reasonable guide the Rings must be precise enough to generate some sort of score, but flexible enough to reflect the fact that deliberation about health care frequently transcends crude counting. The Rings offer the possibility of a basic scoring system which will set limits to their activity. This system must always take the vagaries of life into account – the aspects of care that cannot be effectively modelled. For instance, dependent upon the context it may not always be a disadvantage for a health worker to be standing in the outer circles for the Rings expressed for competence, ethics and law. So to score less than 3, or less than whatever other figure has been selected, need not imply that a halt must be called. In order for a health worker to assess properly whether or not to intervene he must have thought through his priorities; he must be clear about the main theoretical drives of his practice. The primary purpose of the Rings of Uncertainty is not to offer a dubious 'ideal solution' to the question, 'at what point, for how long, and in what way should I intervene?' The Rings are meant to move their users to the point where they recognise it is essential to have a coherent opinion about the importance of their work, and also to offer a logical starting point for the development of such a rationale.

A further educational use

The scoring system can be used to review the past performances of any health worker, as a learning experience, to enable her to consider whether or not she should have practised as she did. Or if this is too threatening the scoring system could be used to assess hypothetical health workers in invented cases.

Three exercises to show the full value of the Rings

16 Using the Rings of Uncertainty fully expressed

Consider this difficult medical situation, and imagine how a doctor might deal with it by employing the Rings as an aid to his deliberation.

Dr Wilson is a consultant paediatrician facing an unpleasant problem. He is responsible for the care of a severely handicapped neonate – a week-old infant. The baby has an inoperable condition but, with prolonged intensive care, stands a 50% chance of surviving, for a few years at least. However, it is likely that his distress – both mental and physical – will be so great that many people would not judge his life to be worth living. The baby's parents – both Catholic – are desperately distressed.

As a general rule Dr Wilson concerns himself only with patients actually in his care. He believes he cannot be expected to consider potential patients as well – even though because of lack of facilities he may have to turn away some who have better chances than his current patients. The doctor is accustomed to dramatic medicine, and often makes 'heroic' interventions. He believes and 'death with dignity' a crucial concept for his branch of medicine, that 'letting die' is fundamentally different from 'killing', and is preferable by far.

However, Dr Wilson is a thoughtful man, inclined to reassess his position periodically. He decides his present dilemma – which is whether or not to continue intensive care for this baby – provides good opportunity for a re-examination of his motives and role. He resolves to picture himself within the Rings of Uncertainty.

The primary issue here is not 'What should I do?', although this is a question he must answer, but 'What is my proper role here? To what extent ought I intervene in this situation? To what extent am I equipped to undertake the various options?'

The Rings expressed

Dr Wilson considers that he needs to use all the available segments: competence, resources, law, communication and ethics. Thus he has an initial picture of the Rings as shown in Figure 40.

Dr Wilson is not sure, before he has thought the problem through, how large each segment should be – so he decides to leave them roughly equal. Even the relative importance of the elements of the problem is uncertain at this stage.

How can Dr Wilson perceive his position? How is he to determine his proper role in this case? What should limit his practice?

Clearly there are several considerations, potential limits and possible courses of action in play. Not all the options will be of the same merit, but he might choose more than one.

Dr Wilson begins to explore the Rings. Logically enough he begins in the competence segment. Now, if Dr Wilson sees himself standing outside the Rings – where he has no special skill or knowledge – he should stop his deliberation at this initial thought. If he is not competent to make the decision he should pass the problem over to someone else, or to a team of people. Perhaps a nurse, a priest, a philosopher or the parents will be better equipped to make the best decision.

In fact Dr Wilson is not so unassuming. He tentatively places himself within the second circle from the centre (B), thus acknowledging that others are expert too. But he is careful not to annul his option to assert his authority, if he thinks it necessary. By picturing himself standing in this part-circle for the Rings expressed for technical competence Dr Wilson has retained the right to continue to reflect about his role. He does not accept that his less-than-perfect

16 Using the Rings of Uncertainty fully expressed   (Continued)

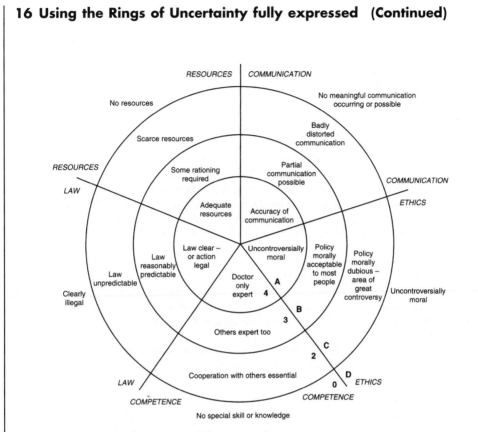

Figure 40 The Rings of Uncertainty fully expressed

competence to make this judgement should limit him. He may not be right, however. He is deliberating only with himself. He may face a tougher test to establish his claim to a role in conversation with others.

He worries about the law. He is profoundly aware of the Arthur case[109] and of Re B.1.[110] As he understands the law, if he were to kill the baby by poisoning him, then he might run the risk of a charge of murder. If he intends active euthanasia, then the law is a serious restriction. But this is not his intention.

Dr Wilson has long held the belief that to discontinue treatment is not a positive act (although not everyone shares this view).[111] For him not doing something is not morally equivalent to doing something. If there were no medical facilities the baby would not be alive in any case. Not to treat is natural, he thinks. Doctors are not 'gods'. Sometimes it is better to 'let nature take its course'. Dr Wilson is also familiar with many precedents for this (he has made similar interventions in the past, and he is reassured that Dr Arthur was not found guilty). However, he recognises some risk of legal action and so places himself in the second innermost Ring (B), since he regards the law as only reasonably predictable.

He knows he ought to involve the parents if at all possible, at the very least to ascertain their wishes. However, there are tremendous problems of communication. Both parents regard life as sacred, but both are also acutely aware of the horrifying condition of their baby. They

(Continued)

16 Using the Rings of Uncertainty fully expressed (Continued)

are crying, grieving already, and their competence to reason calmly is obviously diminished. In addition, it is hard for all concerned to discuss ending the life of such a young and vulnerable being. Consequently, Dr Wilson decides to close up the communication segment, making it comparatively small – he doesn't regard it as particularly important and places himself in the outer circle of the small segment (C) in the belief that communication will inevitably be badly distorted. Dr Wilson also thinks that since he has considered the possibility that the parents might have as much expertise as he does, and has found them to be temporarily incapacitated, he must now see himself as standing within the centre circle for technical competence (A), moving inwards one circle. Only he is expert at this decision now. He feels that if he decides to discontinue treatment (which is his inclination) then it will be important to ensure that the parents do not suffer guilt – he will prevent this burden at least.

At this point Dr Wilson would certainly face a strong challenge from other quarters. He does not have privileged access to some 'moral truth', and it is not out of the question that a stronger justification might be advanced for an alternative policy. However, the purpose of describing a doctor reflecting upon his position within the Rings of Uncertainty is to display the working of the process rather than to advance a moral argument.

Dr Wilson's resources are adequate. He is within the centre circle for this segment – he has time, staff, equipment and finance. Treatment is available for the child, if it is considered appropriate. Afterwards, however, if the baby survives he will continue to need expensive care. Even later there will be a significant demand on state resources to maintain and support the infant.

Dr Wilson looks at the image he has produced and sees he has not only clarified the situation but arrived at a decision. His image looks like this:

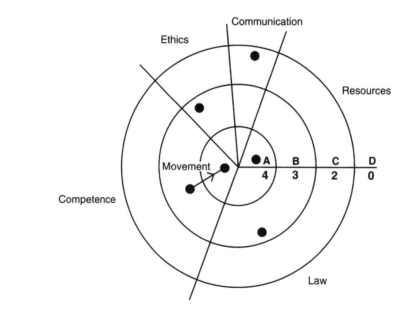

Figure 41 Dr Wilson's picture

16 Using the Rings of Uncertainty fully expressed   (Continued)

According to his personal scoring system the doctor feels he should – in the best interest of the child and his parents – discontinue intensive care. He thinks this would be acceptable to most people, especially if they could witness his deformities and suffering. He realises he does not know this for sure, and is aware that whatever decision he takes will be contentious.

He scores 16 divided by 5, an average score of over 3 – so he is reassured he has a role (which was the major part of his initial question). He is operating within a variety of uncertainties. In addition to his uncertainties of interpretation, of ethics and of self, he does not know what will happen to the child if therapy is discontinued. Dr Wilson is clear, however, that he is operating within the limits of medicine. 'Who else', he asks, 'could take such a decision?'

Other people might place Dr Wilson in different circles, and set the segments to different sizes. However, because Dr Wilson has produced a clear graphic image, because he has made his deliberation about the extent of his role overt and explicit, the use of the Rings at least allows meaningful conversation to start.

The case of the badly handicapped neonate is not one that can have a happy solution. Whatever the decision, there will be tragedy. A more complete ethical analysis would involve a detailed consideration of the range of cost and benefits, a discussion of the doctor's duty and priorities, and an assessment of the severity of the various potential harms (or dwarfings) with a view to minimising them. In other words, a full analysis requires the Ethical Grid.

Exercise

1 Do you agree with Dr Wilson's decision and use of the Rings?

Return to this question once you can use the Ethical Grid competently. Use the Grid to help you deliberate as if you are Dr Wilson.

2 Do you now agree with Dr Wilson's decision and use of the Rings?

17 Live or let die?: uncertainty of role

Consider an emotionally fraught disagreement between two adult offspring about the treatment of their dying mother. The mother is in her eighties. Two years ago she suffered a severe stroke which paralysed one side of her body. Between then and now she has been cared for full-time by her 48-year-old daughter. The son has a home in America, where he works as an engineer.

The mother has contracted pneumonia, and is semi-comatose. On diagnosing the condition the doctor speaks to both son and daughter, outlining the options, which are: do nothing (in which case death is likely in days); treat with antibiotics at home (in which case the infection may clear, though it will probably return shortly); or to treat 'aggressively' in hospital (in which case the infection may be resisted for longer). The daughter, feeling that her mother is no longer 'properly alive', wants no intervention. However, the son wants 'everything possible' done to save his mother.

(Continued)

17 Live or let die?: uncertainty of role   (Continued)

The doctor counsels both offspring, who fail to reach agreement. The doctor then calls in key relatives, including the sister of the sick woman, who eventually persuade the son to concur with his sister.

Setting aside discussion about the morality of euthanasia, the central issue in this case is the role of the doctor. At present her clinical training equips her to diagnose the condition, and prescribe appropriate treatment. It does not, usually, equip her to counsel. It certainly does not legitimise interventions beyond the treatment of disease, and certainly not into the lives of others who have no disease. It is fair to say, 'What else could she do in such a situation?' But it is nonetheless important to recognise the need for clarification of the doctor's role.

Exercise

Consider the limits of the doctor's role by the use of the Rings of Uncertainty fully expressed. Include any further background details you feel necessary – or imagine yourself to be the doctor in question tackling a similar case.

Having thus clarified the situation, analyse it with the benefit of the Ethical Grid, once you have it mastered. What should the doctor have done to create the highest degree of morality?

18 Dealing with dying

If this is to be used for either a role play or exercise then select a character.

The characters

Louise (a woman close to death from cancer)
Daniel (her son)
Dr Jonathan Cook (senior lecturer in oncology – cancer specialist)
Marianne (a SRN on Ward 12)

Louise

Louise is a 48-year-old widow first diagnosed with breast cancer 4 years ago. She underwent a radical mastectomy followed by radiotherapy and chemotherapy. Two years later a recurrence was found in her lymph node. Now a brain secondary has been confirmed. Louise has been admitted to Ward 12, often used to house terminally ill patients, although other people with cancers are also cared for here. Louise has been a patient on this ward three times before.

Louise has not been told explicitly by anyone that she has a brain secondary. However, she feels prepared for death, but has not yet been able to talk about her mortality with anyone in her family other than her sister, with whom she has often stayed during her illness years. She told Dr Cook a few months ago he was not to continue treating her just to keep her alive when things became hopeless.

18 Dealing with dying (Continued)

It is almost Christmas, and the ward is plastered with tinsel, greeting cards and plastic images of Santa Claus. Christmas has a reassuring continuity which Louise thinks is nice. She feels surrounded by other Christmases. Images of her late husband, and a house full of excited children expecting carloads of friends and relatives, pass through her mind.

Louise feels in a daze. She is often confused, and fully lucid only intermittently. When she can make sense she seems to talk more as a little girl than a woman. But this is some sort of defence, helped by her pain-killing drugs. She knows she is dying, and feels indescribably tired, though when she becomes more alert she seems to come back to life. Then she expresses regret at her passivity, she 'doesn't know what came over her', and reasserts her determination to fight, to get better soon. Louise is a chaos of emotions, a cocktail of denial, resistance and acceptance.

When she accepts she can think only of a single wish, which she has not the strength to fulfil. She simply wishes she could tell Daniel she loves him.

Daniel

Daniel is 24, the eldest of Louise's three children. By coincidence he lives close to the hospital where his mother is being treated, while his brother and sister live over 90 miles away. He feels he must somehow assume responsibility as the chief next-of-kin to his mother, and so he visits her every day.

Daniel feels he is a disappointment to his mother. As a youth he was far more interested in having a good time than in study or a career. But he is now in his second year at the local university where he is a mature student. It took a lot of work and self-control to get there and he wishes his mother would acknowledge his recent efforts. He believes (with justification) his mother sees him as 'the bad sheep' – a bit of a waster.

Daniel feels numb. He knows his Mum must die soon, but cannot grasp this as a reality. He cannot picture his mother dying. Looking out of the window of the bus to the hospital each day the world seems more distant than it used to be, as if he were an observer not really taking part in any of it. During his visits the conversation is slow and sparse. Mother and son talk about plants and pets, which are mutual interests, but nothing more important. He feels he would like to express everything he has ever felt for his mother: his anger, his frustration, his need for approval, his sorrow for hurting her, but he cannot even get so far as to think 'I need to tell her I love her'. When he is with her he closes in on himself.

Dr Jonathan Cook

Dr Cook is a senior doctor. He has vast experience of cancer treatment and prognosis, and of the medical care of the dying. He is a hard-working academic and a kind man. Dr Cook thinks Louise is an exceptional patient. He believes that without her determination she would have been dead 2 years ago, but she is a fighter and he knows how important that is in cancer patients.

Dr Cook is also fond of Louise. He is a similar age, and from a similar background. They have had some frank conversations during the treatment programme, but now he feels less able to be open.

He has not thought through the reasons why his attitude has changed, but has withdrawn rapidly from the relationship with the dying woman. He now keeps a 'professional distance' and leaves virtually all the care to the nursing staff. He has, and still has everyday, the opportunity to tell her that she definitely has a brain tumour, and is approaching death. But he doesn't do it. Louise is now under the direct care of a more junior doctor. Dr Cook feels that

(Continued

18 Dealing with dying (Continued)

speaking to Louise is no longer his role. If the other doctor wishes to tell her then that is for him to decide.

Marianne

Marianne hates this ward. She finds it desperately stressful to have to nurse people who are dying and often in great distress. She has applied for a transfer to intensive care where there is at least as much stress, but where people do sometimes recover. Marianne has been nursing Louise for 3 weeks, and is truly torn by the experience. When Louise is lucid and talking of getting better and going home, Marianne feels very close to her. Louise has a sweet nature which reminds Marianne of her own mother. But when Louise is in decline, Marianne just wishes she wouldn't wake up.

Marianne has observed the relationship between Louise and her son, and is familiar with their communication difficulties. She can see they are exceptionally bad at it, and it upsets her.

Marianne is always cheerful on the surface, always the jolly nurse. Daniel scowls at her when he sees her. He thinks her gaiety is quite inappropriate, just like the elaborate Christmas decor. Marianne doesn't know this. She thinks he is an unpleasant and inadequate young man. Why doesn't he just hold his mother's hand for Chrissake?

Marianne has spoken to the social worker to ask her to speak to Daniel. She doesn't feel able to speak to Daniel and Louise herself, though she would dearly like to try to encourage them to talk to resolve their relationship.

The situation

There is a crisis. Daniel has come for an afternoon visit. Louise is drowsy, but conscious. She is lying on her side, breathing wheezily. She seems very warm to Daniel as he leans over her to whisper hello. He is surprised to notice she seems to smell of babies. As he moves to find a chair he spots that her saline drip has gone. He is pleased, he feels a surge of hope. But then he thinks again, as he sits quiet and still. A middle-aged woman in the bed opposite catches his eye, and starts to talk to him.

'Its a shame, its a shame, it really is. She's not very old . . . neither are you. It's a shame. I know her well you know. We were in here together last year. Oh . . . it really is a shame.'

What's she talking like this for? Daniel jumps up in instant fear. He runs to the desk. He asks Marianne what's happening (he doesn't know her name). She says she isn't sure (though she is). Dr Cook has said Louise is not to be disturbed anymore. She's not to have any more medication.

'Where is he? I want to see him. Please.' Daniel is first polite, then begins to shout. 'Where is that bloody doctor? I want him here now. He doesn't know what he is doing. Come on. I'm not leaving until he comes. Please get him here. Get him here.' Becoming increasingly agitated, Daniel leans over the desk and begins to push notes and files to the floor.

Exercise

1 Imagine the situation up to now from the point of view of your selected character. Try hard to imagine the situation from the points of view of other characters.
2 Now act out in your imagination what happens next, playing the part of your selected character. Imagine the situation from the points of view of other characters.
3 If in a class with others, act out the situation as a role play.

What are the main implications of this situation? What should the roles of the doctor and nurse be? What skills might they need?

Using the Rings fully expressed

1 Select a character (either Dr Cook or Marianne).
2 Decide what to do next.
3 Using the Rings fully expressed (Figure 40) place markers/picture yourself within the Rings. If you like, calculate the level of risk of your plan. Remember you can alter the size of the segments.

Examples: Marianne might decide to expel Daniel from the ward. She may attempt to do this herself.

Dr Cook might agree to recommence treatment.

Dr Cook and Marianne might decide to call on others – perhaps including social work staff – for help.

Using the Ethical Grid

Imagine you are Marianne. Devise a strategy to create the highest degree of morality. Criticise your scheme as rigorously as you can, using as much of the Grid as possible.

The Background to the Ethical Grid

Introduction

This chapter explains the thinking behind the Ethical Grid. If you want to use the printed version of the Grid in class, or if you want to understand the assumptions on which the Grid is based, then this chapter is a must-read. If you use or intend to use the Values Exchange (www.values-exchange.com) then you might want to read this chapter out of interest, to learn a little about the philosophical background to the Values Exchange and perhaps to appreciate some of the compromises necessary for the software.

An analogy

The Ethical Grid is not a conveyer belt. It does not deliver correct answers in neat packages – rather it is like a gardener's spade. Like a good gardener, the proficient Grid user understands the importance of keeping her tool clean and sharp. Whether the implement is a spade or the Grid, and whether it is employed on soil or persons, the good worker will recognise when to use it. Sometimes conditions are unsuitable – the ground may be waterlogged, or the law or a social policy clear and agreed (though even in these cases it is worth trying the Grid out, to see what it reveals). Furthermore, the end results of even the most masterful use of either tool are never entirely predictable. Even with the most conscientious practice there is no guarantee that a particular digging method (there is a range of options open to gardeners) will produce the desired horticultural results, and it is equally possible that even the most painstaking use of the Grid may not spawn the best practical results.

What is the Grid and how does it work?

On referring to the figure of the complete Grid (Figure 48) the following features will be noticed:

1 There are four different layers to the Grid, indicated by different colours (blue, red, green and black).
2 Each of the boxes, whatever its colour, is self-contained and detachable.
3 The Grid can be seen in more than one way. It is possible to use it as if the coloured layers have to be addressed in a set order. For instance, a user might think the most significant principles are those contained in the blue boxes at the centre of the Grid, and that the outer boxes are of decreasing importance as one steps (or spirals if that is the preferred method) to the outer limit of the Grid. But this use is not necessarily always the most appropriate.

Alternatively a user might follow a spiral running from the outer limit of the Grid into the blue core, or might always begin with a consideration of consequences, or might always consider – as a start – four specific boxes, one taken from each coloured layer.
The Grid can also be seen as either a two- or three-dimensional object. If it is envisaged in three dimensions the four sides of the pyramid might be considered in turn. However, there is no special relationship or association between the boxes on each side.

4 The Grid has to be applied to practical cases for it to come to life.

Why is the Grid composed of different coloured layers?

First of all it must be explained that the Grid is an artificial device, and the separation of boxes into apparently airtight compartments is also artificial. Nor is it suggested that the Ethical Grid is an exact representation of the mental processes that make up moral reasoning, which is by no means as precise a procedure as the Grid might make it appear. However, in order to provide health workers with a practical and accessible route into moral reasoning, the layers have been distinguished by the use of colour. Given time and experience it ought not be necessary to refer to the Grid at all – it is certainly not a substitute for moral reasoning. Yet even the most seasoned moral thinker might find it useful to refer back to the Grid from time to time, to remind herself of the elements that should be part of a thorough deliberation.
The Grid is presented in four layers to show that at least four aspects are necessary to comprehensive ethical analysis. A deliberation that examines only the consequences of actions, or only the law, or only duties, might happen to produce good results, but it will not have been carried through with integrity. Furthermore, health work deliberations should, if the resulting actions are to be health work at all, refer to at least one box from the blue layer.
It is not suggested that before every intervention the health worker pulls out his 'pocket Ethical Grid' and selects boxes until he is satisfied he has the right combination. This would be quite impractical. Nor is it claimed that the Grid is an indispensable advance in ethical reasoning. But it does make some of the processes of moral reasoning clearer for those unfamiliar with this way of thinking, and as such it is an aid both to understanding and to confidence. The thoughtful health worker can first become familiar with the Grid and its use by practising on hypothetical cases, and then by applying it to cases in practice where there is sufficient time. Proficiency in moral reasoning will improve with practice.

The Ethical Grid has been constructed with health professionals in mind, but it can also be used by people who are not paid to work for health, as its evolution into part of the Values Exchange shows.

The blue layer

The blue layer is set at the centre of the Grid because it is its core rationale. Its four boxes represent – in the most basic manner – the key components of the foundations theory of health.[8,24] The Ethical Grid should be seen as a practical manifestation of this theory (in the form shown in this chapter, but not as it is in the Values Exchange).

Create autonomy

What is autonomy (brief answer)?

Why is the creation of autonomy a central part of work for health? This question may be answered quickly: by focusing on practical tradition, and by studying other theories of health.

The historical tradition
Whatever the means, whether through a personal regime of living or a medical and health professional intervention, practical work for health has always been carried out with the intention of creating autonomy. If treatments are not designed with this end in mind there is little point in making them at all.

A broken arm is a physical impediment to autonomy, and also an obstacle to biological development. Unless it is excruciatingly painful a broken arm does not undermine autonomy completely – a wide range of choices and possibilities will often remain – but it does restrict personal possibility to a degree. An intervention to mend a broken arm is obviously carried out in order to remove the obstacle to normal biological development, but this is not the only reason; it is also carried out in order to enable the person to move on in life without the obstacle. In other words the health intervention is done in order to allow a person the maximum degree of autonomy. The whole point of humane treatment is to enable full persons to flourish as much as possible.

The goal of autonomy has, as a matter of fact, always inspired health work.

All plausible theories of health equate work for health, in some way, with the creation of autonomy
In a previous work[8] a variety of theories of health are presented and discussed. Among the most influential are: the theory that health is an ideal state, the theory that a person is healthy if she can function in a socially useful role, the theory that health can be bought or given as if it is a commodity, and the theory that health is an ability or strength to adapt to the changing challenges and circumstances of life. Though these theories do not share a common view of health, each makes good sense up to a point – and each incorporates the idea of autonomy to some degree. For instance, the World Health

Organisation's 'ideal state' is one in which a person is physically, mentally and socially well, has a satisfying life, and can be economically productive – all notions that require a good level of autonomy. Autonomy is obviously required to carry out a socially useful role (although the level needed will vary dependent upon the role and the society), and the giving or selling of medical commodities – though done for a variety of reasons is nevertheless valuable in direct proportion to the increased autonomy brought about in the receivers or purchasers of the commodities. Finally, the ability to adapt to life's changing circumstances is actually a general definition of autonomy, according to which health just is personal autonomy, and work for health the creation of an ability to thrive (or at least persevere) whatever trauma is suffered.

What is autonomy (detailed answer)?

Several ethical principles have been hailed as health care's primary inspiration. 'Being just', 'not doing harm' and 'doing positive good' are all candidates.[112] At times each can assume temporary precedence over competing notions, even when some forms of autonomy are at stake. For example, when a resource is scarce not all 'autonomy claims' can be met and just distribution must be the priority. Nevertheless, autonomy is the pivotal health care notion.

Autonomy is basic to health care
To say autonomy has no importance in health care is a contradiction in terms:

1 Under Western law consent is essential in any health care intervention that involves touching a competent person. Without consent, touching is a civil or criminal offence. In order for a person to consent to an operation he must have sufficient knowledge to understand the implications of what is proposed. To put it another way, his level of autonomy must be sufficient to give him command of the decision.
2 There is no difference in kind between the problem of disease and other problems of life – there is difference of degree only. All problems affect an individual's autonomy – when a person has a problem her autonomy is lessened by definition, at least in the part of her life where the problem exists. Because disease is not radically different from other problems health workers have no special obligation or right to fight it. Any justification of work against disease must refer to the creation of autonomy, since this is fundamental.
3 Work for health is work to liberate enhancing human potentials. This enhancement is necessarily the creation of autonomy. Health work can diminish only when this diminishing avoids worse harms.
4 Unless an arbitrary distinction is made between physical and mental mobility, if autonomy is a priority then physical and mental autonomy matter equally.

These four points make most sense once a distinction between different understandings of autonomy is grasped. There is Understanding A – *autonomy as being able to do* – and Understanding B – *autonomy as being able to have one's expressed wants*. These categories are explained during the course of this chapter.

Autonomy is not health work's only inspiration. In complicated situations extensive deliberation is required (the Ethical Grid is meant to support precisely this). However, interventions that make no attempt to increase autonomy are not health work.[113]

The richness of autonomy

In most medical ethics literature an 'autonomous person' is said to be 'self-determining' – to have control of her destiny. Autonomy is taken to involve personal wants – an autonomous person can determine what she desires and if her autonomy is respected no-one will stand in her way. But this is Understanding B only. It fails to grasp the depth of autonomy's meaning.

There are at least three different ways of thinking about autonomy.

Autonomy as a single principle

On this understanding autonomy is a principle that 'the wishes of individuals ought to be respected'. Critics of the use of this principle[114] point out that 'autonomy is not the only ethical imperative'. Commentators are quite correct to say that in some circumstances other considerations take precedence over the desires of individuals (for instance, if a person has irrational desires, or if his desires will cause avoidable harm to others) but wrong to believe they have therefore exposed the limitations of the concept. They have not, because autonomy should be thought of more broadly.

The mistaken devaluation of autonomy is common within the pages of some medical journals, particularly in papers on 'ethics in medicine' by doctors who lack philosophical education. For example, a paper in the *Journal of the Royal College of General Practitioners* asked doctors to say what they would do in brief vignettes about control of information in 'unhealthy lifestyle'.[115] The authors chose to offer 'patient welfare' and 'patient autonomy' as contrasting reasons for action. But by separating welfare and autonomy like this the authors assume 'autonomy' means nothing more than 'patient control of decision-making'. If so the only question is does the principle of autonomy apply in this case, or is it better that the doctor decides? Not only is this a very crude representation of clinical reality (where education, conversation, coercion, guilt and recrimination often subtly combine) but it reflects little of autonomy's real meaning. In fact, as we shall see, concern for patient welfare is itself a central part of autonomy creation.

Autonomy as a right

The view that autonomy is a principle has led many writers to claim that autonomy is a right. To assert the right to autonomy is to declare that people capable of self-determination ought not be manipulated, even if others believe this is in their best interest. This is a plausible view of autonomy, but again it is too simple. It regards autonomy as a single type of thing (like life or property – which you either have or have not) which everyone – apart from those whose thought processes are disabled for one reason or another – should have.

This makes perfect fighting sense where people are repressed, where human beings are not allowed self-determination and creative self-expression, and where they might be freed. In such cases to speak of the right to autonomy can be a powerful and emotive weapon. In these circumstances one might justly scream – these people have a right to autonomy! But although this may be politically effective it is impossible to demonstrate that moral rights exist. We have many legal rights, but laws are invented. No-one can show conclusively that 'human rights' exist in any form other than human convention. We do not have an objective right to life, we merely have life.

Despite volumes of writing on the subject,[116] to cast argument for change in rights language is philosophically unhelpful. To speak of autonomy as a right is to do nothing more than to say 'I believe that the human ability to choose should be acknowledged and personal choices respected'. However often this is said, and by however many people, autonomy does not move one jot nearer to becoming an objective right. To speak of autonomy as if it is a right is to perpetuate the myth that autonomy is a single state – something that a person either has or has not – and is something that can be attained or ceded.

Autonomy as a quality

Autonomy is essentially a quality, not a disembodied principle or a right partially separate from human beings. It is utterly wrong to think of autonomy as something that is entirely lost if a right to choose is denied.

Rather autonomy is an intrinsic personal quality. At its most basic, *to be autonomous is to be able to do – to be able to do anything rather than nothing*. Autonomy, thought of in this way, is a matter of degree – the better the level of the autonomy the more a person is able to do. A person becomes able to move more extensively in her life as her level of autonomy rises.

This view of autonomy is more complicated than the other versions, and requires detailed explanation. Much of the rest of this chapter is devoted to this task. By thinking of autonomy as a quality it is possible to move forward on several fronts. It becomes possible to:

1 Make a clear distinction between creating autonomy and respecting autonomy.
2 Show conclusively that respecting autonomy in the sense of 'agreeing to the wishes of others' (a derivative of Understanding B) is a weak idea without reference to the creation or increase of autonomy (Understanding A). When autonomy is conceived of as a basic quality essential to human dignity, which can be enhanced or diminished dependent upon what happens to or is done to people, then work to increase autonomy becomes work to raise the level of human possibility. More prosaically, in a medical context it may be that a doctor considers he is abiding by the principle of autonomy and respecting a patient's right to autonomy in full so long as he is neutral and does not place undue influence upon him. It is not uncommon to hear doctors argue that a

'laissez-faire' approach shows sufficient regard for autonomy – 'the main thing is to let the patient make up her own mind' and 'it's not always up to me to tell the patient everything about his condition – if he wants to know he will ask'. But without additional help this may not be enough – the patient may not have a high enough level of autonomy. Her autonomy may not yet be of a quality good enough to enable her to exercise a reasoned choice.

Indeed, if doctors think respecting autonomy merely means saying 'over to you' whenever there are hard clinical decisions to be made, they have things badly wrong. Superficially it may seem as if a patient's 'right' to exercise the 'principle' is respected if she is left alone to decide to have treatment or not. Certainly she will not be under pressure to do what clinicians would like, but without advice, support and education – and especially if she is upset and anxious – she may have little or no autonomy to exercise.

3 List ways of enhancing autonomy and contrast these to diminishings or constrainings. In this regard it is important to recognise that the quality of autonomy can be improved or worsened by factors internal to a person – factors at least partly within the power of individuals – and external factors too.

4 Demonstrate that in health work there is a crucial point at which efforts to create autonomy (Understanding A) – efforts to improve the quality of a person's autonomy by trying to enhance what that person is able to do – become secondary to a duty to respect autonomy in the sense urged by talk of principles and rights (Understanding B). It can be shown that an autonomy flip can occur, where work to create autonomy must give way to respect for autonomy.

5 Begin to consider solutions to a seemingly intractable dilemma. This occurs whenever it is felt more important to provide for a person's welfare (creating autonomy in line with Understanding A) than to respond to a person's expressed wants (respecting autonomy in line with Understanding B). One trivial example of this dilemma occurs when a decision is made to deny fat children sticky buns even though they want them. A perhaps more serious example confronts doctors who work with people who experience problems with illicit drug use. Should doctors provide the drugs cheaply and safely – which is what many drug users want – or should they insist on detoxification out of concern for their welfare? Which policy has most regard for autonomy?

(Note: It is true to say that if it is argued that autonomy is a quality, and that this quality ought to be increased, then this belief could be translated into a principle. Equally, if health workers have a duty to enhance this quality in others, then it might be argued that this implies a right to have one's autonomy increased.

The first suggestion is undoubtedly true – we create principles and there is no reason why we should not create this one. However, we must remember that the principle is not a thing in itself but originates from admiration of a complex human quality.

The second recommendation is a little more complicated. If it is meant to imply an objective right, then it is wrong. The duty to create autonomy stems from health workers' decisions to commit to work for health, and does not exist before this pledge. Furthermore, a health worker does not have an indefinite duty to create autonomy, but is limited by her understanding of health.)

Autonomy as a human quality

The view that autonomy is a human quality stems from the foundations theory of health mentioned earlier (see p. xii), according to which work for health is supposed to remove obstacles in the way of human potential. Not all of these can be eliminated by cutting away. Some can be removed only through the provision of something else. For instance, ignorance is an obstacle that can be remedied only by giving information. Work for health, thought of in this sense, is work to enable, work to provide a stage on which to perform. The greater a person's stage the more movement in life she will have.

This view of health must explain autonomy as a quality. Because health is directly related to the freedom of body and mind, and not necessarily associated with freedom from disease and illness, autonomy does not just mean the ability of a person to command her physicians. According to the foundations theory of health autonomy makes full sense only when it means being able to do in the widest sense.

There are degrees of autonomy as a quality – it is not something one either has or has not. Autonomy is not, however, necessarily related to the number of options available. Much depends upon context. A physically disabled child living in poverty with an uncaring family – a child living in conditions that disadvantage him on top of his handicap – will have a lower level of autonomy than a physically fit, loved, exceptionally talented Eton schoolboy. However, it does not always follow that wealth, age or fitness are connected to levels of autonomy. For example, a 5-year-old child will not have the same range of options as a 30-year-old middle-class insurance executive – he will not usually be able to do as much as freely – but the child will still be able to exert some control over the aspects of his life that matter most to him. For instance, he will probably be able to choose which toys he plays with, and which books he reads – within a range of options. Realistically, taking account of the different contexts of the two people, their levels of autonomy – the quality of what they might do – can be said to be roughly equivalent.

Whoever we are, whatever circumstances we live under, we are all (unless permanently comatose) able to do some things – able to move freely in some areas of life – and constrained in other aspects. These constraints can be internal to us (for example, limit of talent, limit of will-power) or external (for example, restrictions created by the desires of others, or no resources to allow us to travel widely).

Thus it makes good sense to see autonomy as the ability to do, a quality almost all of us possess to some degree, and a quality that can frequently be enhanced in a great range of ways. This insight shows it is possible to work to increase autonomy without having to be a docile pawn in the game of another person. It is possible to work for autonomy in this broad sense without always having to do what another person requests. And this turns out to be a very important distinction.

Creating autonomy – enhancing the human quality of doing – is basic to health care. It is possible to represent the basic ground of work for autonomy in this way. Autonomy increases as a person moves towards the right of the spectrum.

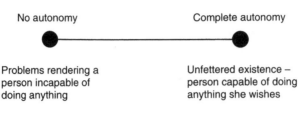

Figure 42 The basic autonomy spectrum

Work to create autonomy does not necessarily imply obedience to patient choice. It is true to say that the creation of choice is a primary goal, but in many cases work can be undertaken to create autonomy without direct reference to it. For example, it may be that a nurse believes a person's depression might be alleviated by a change in his social life. To a withdrawn and lethargic person such a change might not seem at all desirable. However, if the nurse feels change in the person's social life is genuinely worth trying (and the nurse would need to be able to point to evidence to support her proposal) then, in order to create autonomy, she would be justified in a range of attempts to involve the patient in group activity. Although the nurse would not be respecting personal choice immediately, her intent would be to enable the patient to do more, to be freer from the grip of his depression. Hand in hand with the achievement of this goal the patient would gain a higher level of choice. This is not to say that a health worker can force a person to do something against her expressed wishes, but if there is ambivalence then she may seek to create autonomy – but only with the specific aim of moving the person to a position where she is able to exercise a more fully reasoned choice (a choice free from depression in this case). The judgement about the point at which respecting autonomy (Understanding B) must take precedence over creating autonomy (Understanding A) is neither easy nor precisely measurable. Inevitably there will be a grey area in which there will be controversy about whether or not the autonomy flip (see p. 157) has occurred. It is unlikely any foolproof method exists to assist in this judgement, though the Autonomy Test outlined later in this chapter can provide some practical help.

In some cases – where a person is severely mentally handicapped, or where a patient is suffering from a mentally disabling illness – the notion of respect for autonomy may have no part to play. However, this does not mean that the issue of autonomy disappears (as the standard medical ethics account has it). On the contrary, autonomy remains as important as ever. Such a degree of handicap means that a person's life will be subject to some very severe constraints – that the person's autonomy will be of poor quality. If anything, in these cases there is all the more reason to seek avenues that enable the person, even within the severe restrictions of circumstance which surround him. When there is very little of a good thing even the smallest addition can be precious.

In many cases there is a clear relationship between the creation of and respect for autonomy. For instance, it is not possible for a person to express a free wish unless she knows what her situation is, unless she knows the possibilities open to her. So if there are three types of surgery available, and the patient thinks there is only one, she may opt for it, but she will have done so with a lower level of autonomy than she might have

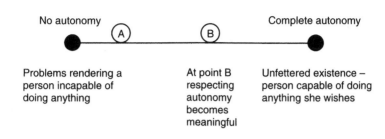

Figure 43 The autonomy spectrum indicating a point of 'autonomy flip'

had. In this way creating autonomy (as enabling mental doing) can be a prerequisite for respecting autonomy (conforming with informed requests).

The fact that wishing depends upon the achievement of a certain level of being able to do – on the provision of certain conditions both for life movement – is even clearer in some other cases. For example, take the case of a frightened, anxious person entering hospital to discuss a future operation. It is possible to be in such a state of nervousness that one cannot think straight. The person may not even be able to comprehend realistically what is being said to him, never mind formulate a coherent view about what to do about his clinical problem. He may, after meeting the consultant in charge, agree to a particular procedure, but since he has not been able to think properly it makes very little sense to say this is what he wants. In order to have any autonomy (on Understanding B) to respect, autonomy (as being able to do – Understanding A) must be raised to a sufficient level. Looked at with reference to the continuum illustrated in Figure 42, the primary task of the health worker is to ensure that the anxious patient moves from A to B on the spectrum (Figure 43).

As a general guide, the impetus of all health care interventions should be first to try to move a person as far to the right of the spectrum as possible, and secondly to move a person past point B on the spectrum at the earliest possible opportunity. Although the exact position of point B is bound to be the subject of some controversy, and must be decided with reference to the particular facts of the case, this does not invalidate the guiding idea.

It must be said that not all health professionals think of their work like this. Those who do not are not working for health on the foundations theory. It is, to be sure, easier and often more efficient not to work as the first priority to move a person from A to B. For one thing the attempt is likely to be time-consuming. But if autonomy is seriously considered an essential goal of work for health, the effort must be made.

Two cases

Consider the following two cases. Both involve consent, although in subtly different ways. Consent might be defined as an expressed agreement to a procedure based on a level of information that would be sufficient to satisfy the giver of that information if he were to be on the receiving end. Bear in mind that consent must be based ultimately in autonomy as ability to do. That is, a person must already be at a certain point on the autonomy spectrum to be able to consent.

---

19 Carole

Think about Carole, an unemployed, unhappy young women. She is living in an apparently close middle-class family, which has profound tensions below the surface. Her father is terminally ill.

Carole's behaviour consists of intermittent lethargy, drunkenness and rebellion – but overall she is catastrophically miserable. She gets in trouble with the law, caught shop-lifting a skirt from Marks and Spencer. Carole's parents decide enough is enough, and she is persuaded to see a psychiatrist, who makes a diagnosis but does not tell Carole or her parents what it is. All he will say is that she has an emotional problem she can be helped with. After a couple of weeks in hospital as a 'voluntary patient' Carole is treated as an outpatient. She is given an injection of a long-lasting anti-psychotic drug (Modecate) and also another drug (Kemadrin procyclidine) to counteract possible 'Parkinsonian side-effects'. She is not told what to expect by either the doctor or the nurse who administers the injection.

There are two key issues to consider in this case. *Does Carole give meaningful consent to her treatment, and in which direction is she moved along the autonomy spectrum?* These questions are crucial in the great majority of health care interventions. Before considering answers in Carole's case consider a little more detail. She is having many difficulties in her life, and clearly at a low ebb. Carole is immensely vulnerable. She is blamed by her family and some of her friends for causing most of her troubles – 'Everybody has problems, why does it always have to be you who over-reacts and makes things even worse?' For her own part she blames herself entirely for her calamity.

Carole desperately wants to be happier, to resolve this situation in which she is drowning. She is an intelligent young woman but drifted away from school before taking her final exams – for which she had not worked anyway. Carole has not studied or read anything other than the tabloid newspapers for the last 3 years: she can't be bothered to read anything else, she can't concentrate and can't see the relevance of any of it to her.

Carole becomes a 'voluntary patient' because she sees it as a way out. She has to do something to get out of the hole and she doesn't have many options left. In addition the pressure placed on her by her family is becoming ever more unbearable. She says she agrees to the drug treatment but she has very little idea what it will do to her, indeed whether it will benefit her in any way (although she knows the demonstration of compliance with her family's wishes might).

The point of this example is not to criticise psychiatry but to show how a lack of a theory of health can diminish autonomy (although something very close to this situation actually happened to me). There were clearly many other ways in which Carole's life might have been enhanced, even if the diagnosis had been correct. When disease, or at least perceived disease, is regarded as the priority, above other problems which might receive attention, then it is inevitable that other ways of improving a person's life will neither be spotted nor pursued.

20 Evelyn

The next example is again taken directly from life. It is discussed towards the end of this chapter and presented now as an exercise for self or group learning.

Research for health?

This case is based on the experience of Evelyn Thomas. Her words have been extracted from an article that appeared in *The Observer* (UK). The report of the feeling and motivation of the chief researcher are imaginary. The justification offered by the actual researcher can be found in the same newspaper.[117]

This exercise describes the feelings of two characters. The situation is that a woman who has had a mastectomy has discovered that she has been involved in clinical trials without her consent. The *first trial*, which took place simultaneously in different centres around Britain, involved the testing of preventive hormonal treatment. Evelyn's treatment was compared with that of other women cancer sufferers who were receiving either no further treatment or different drugs.

The *second trial* was to test the effects of post-operative counselling. Evelyn was not counselled yet other patients were. Their 'psychological adjustment' was compared.

We might call the doctor Alan Hughes since the position for which he argues is not unique to the researcher in question. The view advanced below is a paraphrased amalgam of the beliefs of several doctors. It is not intended to represent accurately the opinion of the Professor in real life.

Dr Hughes explains:

I have been a clinical researcher and consultant surgeon for over 20 years now, and been in medicine for 10 years before that. My experience allows me to balance, in the broadest perspective, long-term human gain against possible short-term individual suffering. I would emphasise my choice of the word 'possible'. The whole point of research is that the answer is not known. It may turn out that the subject of a controlled trial might have benefited more from a treatment from which she was excluded, but equally she might not have done. We simply do not know for sure, which is why we need to experiment.

I know that this patient, and you could say the same of others in the past, feels hurt and perhaps abused by what I have done, but I stand by my actions and refuse to change my practice. If this patient had been informed that she was in either trial it would have rendered her inclusion scientifically invalid. We do not know the precise relationship between mental state and physical well-being, and this might have affected our results. This is particularly obvious in the case of the post-operative counselling. We were searching for very specific information, and only this information. This made it necessary for us to control as many variables as possible.

I think there are three main points to consider here: first of all each research proposal has to be passed – approved – by an ethics committee. These are committees made up of highly experienced, eminent, honourable people. Ethics committees make sure that no research proposal that is at all unethical is passed. They did not consider that I needed consent for my research because they weighed up the costs and benefits, and appreciated the considerable amount of good that potentially could be achieved by the work.

This raises the second point: if clinical research is permitted only if patients are informed, then we would not have the benefit of many scientific advances. It is vital that we advance our scientific understanding for the benefit of all future patients, and any of us might be future patients. It must also be said that most people included in research

(Continued)

20 Evelyn (Continued)

trials do not suffer. In this case no worse treatment was given to the patient. We believed that both drug treatments were roughly equivalent.

As for the counselling trial, the patient received the highest standard of care possible from our doctors and nursing staff. It is true to say that she did not receive this particular form of intervention – but at the time we had no idea whether she would benefit from it or find it to her disadvantage. In any case different people respond in different ways to all forms of medical treatment: medicine is the most uncertain of all sciences – there are always exceptions to all forms of treatment, always people who recover when they seem to have no chance of doing so.

It is also very pertinent to consider what it means to be working at this level in medicine. I cannot just sit still and rest on my laurels. I have to achieve, I have to compete. Some of my younger colleagues – men still in their forties – have published over 300 scientific papers and I have just over 150. I am ambitious and it is expected of me – it is an integral part of the profession that I am involved in. It is unrealistic to expect me to stop doing what so many of my peers are doing: it is part of the profession. Why should I challenge this practice, especially since I regard it to be morally quite justified?

Evelyn Thomas explains her point of view. These are her own words as reported in *The Observer*:

When I was found to have breast cancer I had high expectations of the medical profession. Like most patients I believed the doctors observed strict ethical codes. I placed absolute trust in those treating me and assumed that our relationship was based on openness and frankness. I assumed that my treatment was the only option.

I now know that I assumed too much. Patients with breast cancer presenting themselves to my surgeon in the early 1980s had their treatment determined, without their consent, by computer randomisation. My consultant's role was to diagnose, establish eligibility for entry into clinical trials, withhold information, ensure randomisation, hereafter monitor progress. My rights to have information and to choose, and my responsibility for my own body were denied. My trust was abused I am both deeply hurt and bitterly disappointed to have been so misused by members of the medical profession.

In retrospect, the first indication that I was in a trial came a few days after my mastectomy. The mastectomy patient in the next bed had been seen by a counsellor and given helpful information. The counsellor avoided me, and a breast prosthesis was given to me by a male fitter more used to fitting artificial limbs.

It took several years to obtain confirmation that I had been in a trial. The first trial compared post-operative counselling with no counselling – the availability of counselling was not mentioned to those randomised not to receive it.

The second trial compared three chemotherapy regimes and no treatment; the regimes were tamoxifen tablets, cyclophosphamide injections and a combination of both. Patients were again randomised – to one of the four choices – without any alternative being offered.

The administrators at the hospital had confirmed that I was entered into these two trials without my knowledge. Since a trial of lumpectomy versus mastectomy was also in progress at that time I suspect that I may have been in that trial since I was offered no alternative to mastectomy.

I believe that these trials were wrong for several reasons. At the very least they were unkind. It is unkind not to offer available alternatives to total breast amputation; it is unkind not to offer available counselling to all patients following breast surgery; and it

20 Evelyn   (Continued)

is unkind not to offer to patients an alternative to cyclophosphamide with its side-effect of hair loss that is dreaded.

Withholding information about the trials may also have invalidated them. It was forgotten that patients, unlike laboratory animals, can move around and communicate with each other. Treatments are discussed and unexplained differences discovered. Inevitably these cause worry, and patients may become confused and resentful. Such feelings, and the stress produced, may be the very factors that affect health and well-being.

Secret trials demean patients. By depriving patients of opportunities to make informed choices, doctors appear to assume that we are unintelligent, immature and irresponsible.

Finally, I believe that such trials are unethical. I agree with the principles laid down in the Nuremburg Code for experiments on humans, which state that 'the voluntary consent of the human subject is absolutely essential' and that the person involved 'should have sufficient knowledge and comprehension of the elements of the subject matter involved as to enable him to make an understood and enlightened decision'.

Some doctors violate these ethical principles. They argue that patients cannot cope with full knowledge or uncertainties in its treatment, so that it is kinder to say nothing. Such arguments are wrong, because it is the patient or family who has to cope with an incurable and progressive disease.

I am not arguing against scientific medical research or randomised clinical trials (RCTs). As a patient I have the most to gain from progress. As a scientist who has herself carried out physiological research on human subjects, obviously I approve of scientific methods in medicine. But RCTs must only be used with the informed consent of the participating patients. If investigators cannot convince patients that each arm of an RCT carries equal chance of risks or benefits then they must respect those patients' decisions not to participate.

My experience shows that doctors can no longer assume that secrecy in their dealings with patients can remain undetected. Yet once I did start asking questions of my consultant and hospital, the response continued to be secretive. Relevant questions about my treatment have been met with prevarication and half-truths. Approaches to various organisations such as the Community Health Council and the General Medical Council have produced little progress in getting the information, explanation and discussion that I sought. Indeed the only advice offered by the President of the GMC was that I should take legal action – a sorry reflection on the body that has a statutory duty to control the conduct of doctors.

It is good practice for such trials to be authorised before they start by the hospital's ethical committee, to see whether they are ethically acceptable. The existence of these secret trials therefore raises awkward questions about the committee's role. A letter I received last year from an administrator at the hospital said that informed consent had initially been required for the comparative trial of chemotherapy, but that after a few months the ethical committee had changed its mind. The administrator explained why:

'The reasons for this decision were that the study was being carried out on a national and European level and that other participants on the trial had not felt it appropriate to seek informed consent because of the specifically humane treatment offered in each of the arms of the study. More importantly, the experience nationally and locally was that many patients found it intensely stressful to have to face up to not only consenting

(Continued)

20 Evelyn (Continued)

to mastectomy but very shortly afterwards to have to consider the true nature of their disease and the uncertainty surrounding its management. The decision-making involved in getting informed consent was considered harmful for the welfare of some patients.'

Such reasons are not adequate to explain why the ethical committee chose to ignore the Nuremburg Code and many subsequent guidelines on the ethical conduct of research.

Evelyn Thomas's argument was first published anonymously by the *Bulletin of the Institute of Medical Ethics*.

Exercise

Either imagine that you are Doctor Hughes – and that you have read Evelyn's account – and a junior colleague asks you to lead a new research project which requires the diseased patients to be ignorant that they are subjects of research.

Or imagine that you are Evelyn and the information has been leaked to you by a sympathetic hospital worker that the research has been proposed, and that it has been put to Dr Hughes that he might like to become involved in it.

Where might Dr Hughes picture himself within the Rings?

Imagine that the doctor and Evelyn both know how to use the Ethical Grid. Imagine a conversation between the two, with a Grid on a table between them. How do you think the discussion would go?

Misunderstanding the importance of autonomy

The above example shows a doctor placing other values above both the promotion of individual autonomy and respect for choice. There is little question that the motives of researchers in such cases are complex, and often honourable in that the work is directed towards a general increase of human good. But their research is misguided (according to my view of health and my personal moral commitment) because the importance of autonomy is underestimated.

In the example the researchers place the notions of not causing harm (referring to the stress that might be caused to patients by asking them if they consent to being in a medical experiment), patient welfare (in the sense of not unnecessarily impeding the attempted clinical cure) and the well-being of future patients (who will presumably be helped by advances in the understanding of drug therapies) above that of autonomy (understood in either way – A or B). But while it is right to say that autonomy should not always be the primary health care drive, it should not be overridden so lightly. However politically pleasing many might find the view that medicine should work essentially with communities it remains a fact that individuals suffer the disabling problems we call diseases, and that a doctor works most closely with individual patients. Consideration of patient autonomy (in the broadest sense) must always be the starting point for interventions that seek to work for health.

This was obviously not the case in the above example. Three further errors were committed by the medical professor. Briefly, the first was to think of autonomy as a single principle, the second was to commit a 'category mistake' (wrongly supposing that work for health is the natural concomitant of work to counter disease) and the third was to have left Evelyn at a point unnecessarily near the left of the autonomy spectrum when he might – without harm to anybody else – have moved her further to the right. The professor was not working for health in this case. No genuine health work can regard people only as means, even if they are thought to be means towards greater ends.

The autonomy flip

Before the Autonomy Test is outlined it is important to consider how the notions create and respect autonomy might be ranked in order to guide practical interventions.

Ranking ideas within autonomy

By attempting to rank these two ideas, an apparently unyielding health care dilemma is again brought to the fore. It is this: to what extent should a person's welfare (autonomy as 'being able to do' – Understanding A) take precedence over a person's wants (autonomy as 'being able to have one's choices' – Understanding B)?

Should welfare ever take precedence over wants? All experienced health carers will be familiar with the frustration of watching a person do something to himself that the health carer thinks is foolish, or tragic, or just 'bloody stupid'. Perhaps the person is eating too much or too little, smoking, drinking, engaging in unprotected sex with several partners or injecting heroin. If the person is indulging in any of these habits, a concerned health carer might well consider that this is not good for him – that it cannot possibly be in his interest even though he thinks it is. Understandably a health worker might think it his task to ensure the person changes his ways.

In such cases there can be a strong temptation for some doctors to be paternalistic – in other words for doctors to give their perception of the person's welfare (often referred to as 'health') a higher priority than his choice.

Such a policy assumes this ranking of the two notions of autonomy:

FIRST: CREATE AUTONOMY
SECOND: RESPECT AUTONOMY

The expression create autonomy refers to basic work to enable a person (Understanding A), work to provide adequate conditions of welfare – conditions for a way of life where a person is able to realise fulfilling possibilities. For instance, educating a person about the effect of medication on her body, and ensuring that an extremely stressed person takes a rest, are both actions that would qualify as work to create autonomy.

'Create autonomy' ought to take precedence over 'respect autonomy' when a person clearly faces disabling problems, and makes no objection to the health worker addressing these problems. However, at a point which varies – dependent upon circumstances and the individuals concerned – the two notions 'flip over' like this:

FIRST: RESPECT AUTONOMY
SECOND: CREATE AUTONOMY

The ultimate aim of work to create autonomy is to move a person to a position where she is so unfettered that she is able to exercise an informed choice about what she would like, and able to get it. It is self-evident that:

> Education for health is work for wholeness. It is not just to do with physical functioning, it is at least equally to do with the mental life of a person . . . work for health in its full and proper sense is work towards laying the foundations for full human flourishing.[8]

Human beings are distinguished from most animals by our facility to think – to reflect, to introspect, to plan our actions. Not to pay particular attention to this human asset when working for health is absurd.

The central ethical problem in health care occurs when a carer wants to carry on creating autonomy (as welfare) while the subject believes he has reached a level of autonomy sufficient to permit a reasoned choice, and wants his autonomy respected. This may mean that the subject wishes to have further autonomy created, but in a way unacceptable to the health worker.

Consider a case from practice. Take the example of a person said to be 'abusing heroin'. While 'create autonomy' is ranked first, the health worker can justifiably seek to push the person to the right of the spectrum. So, if the drug-taker seeks help whilst intoxicated the health worker might offer facilities for treatment, might educate about the risks of heroin injection, might counsel, might review the person's life circumstances to see if a changed life-style might be preferable (and possible) as an alternative to heroin-taking, might show the safest ways of injecting, and might argue for whatever point of view she believes in (so long as she does not present this as the only worthwhile possibility, and so long as she does not take advantage of the person's vulnerability to put forward propaganda).

However, once the autonomy flip has occurred work to create autonomy can continue but must always be implemented so as to take the fullest possible account of the wishes of the subject of health care. So, if the drug-taker says something to this effect, 'I have listened to all you have to say, I have learnt from you, but I do not wish to stop my habit, and I do not wish you to try to make me stop anymore', and it is clear that he has the capacity to understand and has made an informed choice, then this wish must be respected.

Of course the duty to respect autonomy is not absolute in all cases. For instance, it is inappropriate if a parent insists 'I wish to continue inflicting unnecessary suffering on my children'. Autonomy ought not be respected if a person's choice will deliberately harm others, and the harm is avoidable. Equally, it might be the case that a health worker has to take wider considerations into account, that to respect individual autonomy in all cases might be to go against what might loosely be described as the 'public interest' (perhaps if the doctor were not to report a chronic epileptic patient seen driving a car).

Neither is it an implication of a commitment to respect autonomy that whatever a person wishes should be provided. It does not follow that because a patient wants ampules of heroin on prescription a doctor has a duty to oblige. But what is implied is that once choice is possible, once the human faculty of reason is present, then the doctor should not positively prevent this choice unless respecting the wish would cause harm to others, or seriously undermine the subject's welfare and the subject does not recognise this.

The Autonomy Test

The Autonomy Test applies only to health care and only to individuals.

In the arena of urgent practice, images and models may seem nothing more than a diversion from reality. Such decision-making tools require time to think through and apply, and this time is not available to most health workers. If Paradigm Y is not to remain an optimistic hope, something immediately applicable is needed.

On many occasions in health care decisions have to be made quickly, even though there are no simple rules available. What is required in these circumstances is a 'litmus test', a speedy way of obtaining a provisional indication whether a proposed course of action ought to go ahead or not, or if it ought to be modified.

Although many health care decisions are perennially debatable, some policies are clearly wrong (according to my Ethics B). The Autonomy Test is of most value in its ability to help expose these cases. It also helps to clarify options for creative progress by focusing on practical ways of moving a person to the right of the autonomy spectrum.

What is the Autonomy Test?

The Autonomy Test is a basic means of checking the appropriateness of plans, and of 'brainstorming' for better possibilities for care. However, the Autonomy Test is also a result of a systematic account of the nature of health, and to use it is to concede many implicit assumptions.

The Autonomy Test – annotated

The Autonomy Test consists of a number of simple questions, and requires a doctor simply to list various possibilities.

One

Will physical or mental autonomy not be increased when it might have been? Will it be diminished in any way?

(Continued)

The Autonomy Test – annotated (Continued)

This is a very demanding question. Only rarely in the context of medical interventions will it be possible honestly to answer *No* to this question. It is very strict. The question requires that if a drug is prescribed with 'side-effects' which diminish, or a person has to stay in hospital, then the response must at this stage be *Yes*. If there is doubt about whether or not an intervention is one that acts to diminish then, if possible, seek the opinion of the subject.

If the answer is genuinely *No* then go to Six. If the answer is *Yes*, or if there is any possibility that it might be *Yes* because a factor has been overlooked, then go to Two.

Two

List the way(s) in which autonomy will be increased and the way(s) in which autonomy will be diminished by the proposed action:

Increases in autonomy   *Diminishings of autonomy

*Note: At this point it is inevitable that there will be disagreement about what things count as increases (enablings) and what as decreases of autonomy (diminishings). It is likely that there will be particular debate over the question of long-term and short-term autonomy. Some will take the view that although autonomy (either in the sense of being able to have wishes fulfilled, or in the sense of being able to move unfettered) is diminished in the short term, this is justified by the probable long-term increase. (This position is sometimes asserted when people are detained – in their perceived best interests – under Mental Health Acts.)

Three

Are each of these diminishings absolutely necessary?
If *No*, then stop. Reconsider the proposed action. Consider a fresh policy.
    If *Yes*, then go to:

Four

Will these diminishings have the effect of increasing the autonomy of the patient (according to either Understanding A or B) in the future?
If *No*, then stop. Reconsider the proposed action. Consider a policy that might work for health instead.
    If *Yes*, then go to:

Five

Are the patient's reasoned wishes being overridden?
If *No*, and the intent is to move the person to the right of the autonomy spectrum as soon as possible, then proceed to Six.
    If *Yes*, then either stop – the 'category mistake'[27] will be committed if disease is challenged at the expense of human choice – or show how this overriding of reasoned wants can be justified in another way. Possible justifications might include:

The Autonomy Test – annotated   (Continued)

1 The individual's wishes will harm me or others unnecessarily
2 The individual is reasoning erroneously – he may be thinking illogically – he may be deriving false conclusions, or he may have false beliefs (but, if so, then an attempt must be made to move him as soon as possible to the point where the autonomy flip can occur).

Note: At this point in the Autonomy Test it is very important to bear in mind the distinction between physical autonomy – the freedom that a person has to live without physical obstruction – and mental autonomy – the freedom that a person has to make decisions and act on them. It is usual for short-term physical autonomy to be decreased in health care in order to increase long-term physical autonomy – restraining an arm in a sling, or prescribing drugs that cause drowsiness in order to cure infections, or injuring a person during surgery: all these are reductions in short-term physical mobility. So long as these diminishings are not imposed against a person's wishes, they are not problematic. But here the insidiousness of the category mistake becomes truly apparent. Although it is a genuine mistake which implies no intent to harm, the mistake can be dangerous. It is one thing to stop a broken leg moving by slapping plaster of Paris around it, yet quite another to prevent a person acting on her choice to drink 'too much' or to have 'too many boyfriends', by classifying her as ill and administering long-lasting tranquillisers. The reduction of mental autonomy, even in the short term with the goal of promoting long-term gain, is far harder to justify in the case of any rational person (whether child or adult) who can understand the implications of what she proposes to do.

Justifications have been attempted, but they smack of miserliness of spirit – just as a financial miser will be forever saving, waiting just a little longer until he spends. For example, it has been argued that breaking a confidence (in other words not respecting a person's choice) is justified so long as this results in greater autonomy for that person in the long term. But it is hard to see the purpose of this. If the person is in a position to choose, then he should be permitted this. Otherwise, on the next occasion that the person with the power to deny choice disagrees with that choice, she will be able to justify its denial by saying that the patient is not yet autonomous enough.

What such an argument basically says is this: although you do have the capacity to choose for yourself, either you are making the wrong choice deliberately, or you cannot see that by making this choice you are shutting a great many doors that would otherwise be open to you. Thus, for the sake of your future capacity to choose – which should be as great as possible – I override your present capacity – and I do it for your sake.

Naturally many kind and experienced people do pursue policies such as this with those they feel could benefit from their 'hidden' support. However, it is always open to such well-meaning closet paternalists to explain in the fullest possible terms why they believe that the other person is making a mistake. There is the danger that since there is no theoretical cut-off point – no binding rule to tell the paternalist when he has gone too far, or continued for too long – that he will, using exactly the same justification time and time again, continue to override personal choice.

The Autonomy Test is clear on this. To satisfy the Autonomy Test the flip should occur just as soon as the person can weigh up the problem, review the options and assess the implications. A free society does not wait until some ideal inspired moment – people must be free to make mistakes.

Six

Consider the list of the ways in which autonomy might be increased (the ways in which latent enhancing human potentials might be made actual). Decide, if at all possible in partnership

(Continued)

The Autonomy Test – annotated (Continued)

with the patient, the order of priority in which this list of possible potentials might be achieved.
    Weigh these against any potential costs.

Seven

Once decided and agreed – initiate proposed action.

The Autonomy Test – unannotated

One

Will physical or mental autonomy not be increased when it might have been? Will it be diminished in any way?
If the answer is genuinely *No*, then go to Six.
    If the answer is *Yes*, or if there is any possibility that it might be *Yes* because a factor has been overlooked, then go to Two.

Two

List the way(s) in which autonomy will be increased and the way(s) in which autonomy will be diminished by the proposed action:

Increases in autonomy   **Diminishings of autonomy**

Three

Are each of these diminishings absolutely necessary?
If *No* then stop. Reconsider the proposed action. Consider a fresh policy.
    If *Yes*, then go to:

Four

Will these diminishings have the effect of increasing the autonomy (according to either Understanding A or B) of the patient in the future?
If *No* then stop. Reconsider the proposed action. Consider a policy which might work for health.
    If *Yes* then go to:

Five

Are the patient's reasoned wishes being overridden?
If *No*, and the intent is to move the person to the right of the autonomy spectrum as soon as possible, then proceed to Six.
    If *Yes*, then either stop – the *category mistake* will be committed if disease is challenged at the expense of human choice – or show how this overriding of reasoned wants can be justified in another way. Go to Six.

The Autonomy Test – unannotated   (Continued)

Six

Consider the list of the ways in which autonomy might be increased (the ways in which latent enhancing human potentials might be made actual). Decide, if at all possible in partnership with the patient, the order of priority in which this list of possible potentials might be achieved.
   Weigh these against any potential costs.

Seven

Once decided and agreed – initiate proposed action.

Applying the Autonomy Test

Although the Autonomy Test is crude and open to interpretation, it is nevertheless a guideline that health workers might choose to adopt. It is enlightening to apply the test to various cases in real life. This will usually give clear answers. It is not necessary to go into detailed ethical analysis of most of these cases since the Autonomy Test makes no claim to depth – it is a litmus test, a traffic light: should I stop or should I go? For instance, if Carole's case (see p. 152) is put to the Autonomy Test there is a swift result.

The test applied – Carole

One

Will physical or mental autonomy not be increased when it might have been? Will it be diminished in any way?
Answer: Yes, unequivocally Carole is an intelligent and able girl, yet she does not have enough information about her diagnosis and her treatment. Perhaps even more importantly no work is being done to help her *picture* what is happening to her, to help her conceive of the set of unfortunate circumstances which currently surround her – to help her map out her world Carole desperately needs to recognise that all her problems are not her fault, that failure is just one map out of several possibilities, and that all maps have routes into each other – we can and will all fail at some things.

Two

List the way(s) in which autonomy will be increased and the way(s) in which autonomy will be diminished by the proposed action.
In the case of Carole there have been a series of actions which have dwarfed her unnecessarily. Consider the effect of applying the *Autonomy Test* prior to drug therapy. (Note: not increasing autonomy where it would be possible to do so is taken to be diminishing.)

(Continued)

The test applied – Carole   (Continued)

Increases in autonomy	Diminishings in autonomy
Possible alleviation of psychotic symptoms	Things done to Carole without her understanding
	Family not involved in any therapy
	No counselling – no picturing for Carole
	No attempt to help Carole to find a purpose in her life

Three
Are each of these diminishings absolutely necessary?
Answer: No. Reconsider the proposed action. Consider a fresh policy.

Exercise

Apply the Autonomy Test to the example highlighted by Evelyn Thomas. Address this proposal: Dr Hughes wants to carry out an identical research programme on human subjects. Consider your response with reference to one of the potential subjects, Pauline Johnson.

Limitation of the Autonomy Test

There is much that the Autonomy Test cannot do. There are many cases where what counts as an increase or decrease in autonomy is too open to interpretation for the test to be decisive. To resolve such cases more extensive ethical analysis is necessary, although the Autonomy Test will hardly ever be entirely redundant. For instance, consider the following difficult case.

LAW REPORT

Sterilisation of mental patient not unlawful

A sterilisation operation on a mentally disabled adult patient is not unlawful by reason only of the patient's inability to consent if it is carried out in the best interests of the patient.

The facts

F., who was born in 1953, has the verbal capacity of a 2-year-old and the general mental capacity of a 4- to 5-year-old. She has been a voluntary in-patient at a hospital since 1967, where she has formed a sexual relationship with a male mental patient. The evidence was that she had physical enjoyment from sexual intercourse with him and that she was not being sexually molested.

F. has the fertility of any other woman of her age, and her mother applied for a declaration that it would be lawful for F. to be sterilised, notwithstanding that she was incapable of

Figure 44 The blue boxes

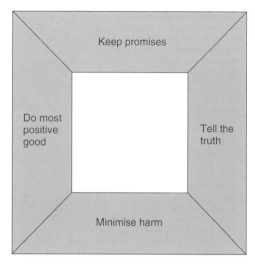

Figure 45 The red boxes

Figure 46 The green boxes

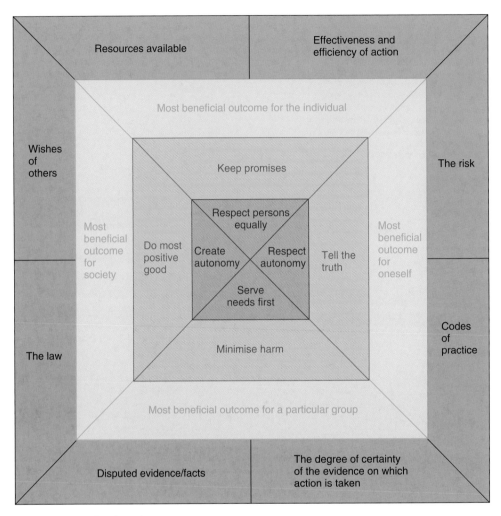

Figure 48 The Ethical Grid

consenting. Mr Justice Scott-Baker granted the declaration (*Guardian Law Report* 3 December 1988). The Official Solicitor, who was given leave to intervene, appealed.

The decision

Lord Donaldson referred to the case of Re B[1988]AC199 in which the House of Lords held that in the case of a mentally handicapped minor the court could, acting in its wardship jurisdiction, consent to the sterilisation of the minor if it was in her best interests. This raised the stark issue of whether the law treated adults who suffered from a disability differently, and on one view less favourably, than it treated children suffering from a similar disability. In the absence of consent all, or almost all, medical and surgical treatment of an adult is unlawful, however beneficial such treatment might be.

F.'s disability was such that she would never be mentally competent to appreciate the issues involved and to consent to sterilisation or to any medical treatment. The court had no power either under the *parens patriae* jurisdiction or under any statutory jurisdiction to dispense with F.'s consent or to give consent on her behalf.

The common law right of body inviolability save with consent was subject to two exceptions: first, emergency medical treatment and, second, physical contacts which are inevitable or at least are a usual feature of everyday life, such as the jostling on public transport, or generally acceptable standards of conduct. A doctor faced with an unconscious accident patient is lawfully entitled and probably bound to carry out such treatment as is necessary to safeguard the patient's life and health, although the patient is in no position to consent.

It would therefore not be surprising if the common law rule were subject to a further qualification in relation to those who by reason of disability are unable to consent. There is a clear and logical connection between the position of an adult who through an accident is temporarily deprived of the power of consent – the emergency treatment case – and the case of an adult who through permanent disability is equally unable to consent. The difference is largely, although not entirely, one of scale.

But the law should not regard adults as permanent emergency cases. In an emergency a doctor had little time but in this case the doctor had more time, and far more was required of him.

The test that the court did, and the reasonable adult should, apply was, 'what course of action is best calculated to promote my true welfare and interests'. What constituted true welfare and interests often gave rise to very difficult questions, but that did not affect the validity of the test.

Lord Justice Neill said the answer lay in considering the public interest. Provided that the operation was necessary within properly defined limits and appropriate safeguards were prescribed, there was no reason in principle why a patient who could not give consent should be deprived of the right to receive the treatment required.

'Necessary' in that context meant that which a general body of medical opinion in the particular specialty would consider to be in the best interests of the patient in order to maintain his health and secure his well-being. Unanimity was not required, but it should be possible to say of an operation which was necessary in the relevant sense that it would be unreasonable in the opinion of most experts in the field not to make the operation available to the patient.

Lord Justice Butler-Sloss concurred.

The appeal was dismissed, and leave was granted to appeal to the House of Lords.[118]

The problem for the Autonomy Test in these circumstances is that the autonomy flip can never occur. F. will never be able to have a sufficient level of autonomy created for her to enable her to consider her situation, and to express a wish.

The judges decided to apply a 'best interests test', but what one person might consider to be in her 'best interests', another might not. For example, a critic of the judgement argued:

> There are a number of deeply disturbing features about this case. It is not clear that the court had the jurisdiction to make the order that it did. And it is not clear that the order made was legally correct. To equate the sterilisation operation, as the judge did, with the extraction of a tooth, the repair of a hernia or the administration of an injection, fails to recognise the enormity of the invasion and injury which the proposed sterilisation represents. It fails to distinguish between the obvious therapeutic advantages in the supposed analogies and the dubious benefits which sterilisation offers. And it fails to acknowledge that sterilisation involves major abdominal surgery requiring general anaesthesia.
>
> As troubling, however, are the assumptions being made about the sexuality of women with a mental handicap, the risks to which pregnancy exposes them, and the response of courts to the interests of what the judge in one place calls 'mental defectives'.[119]

For the judges and the author of this quote the list of increases and diminishings is not the same. A judgement has to be made about who gives the most appropriate list in regard to the creation of F.'s autonomy, and this is not finally decidable. An analysis deeper than the Autonomy Test is required for this, but at least the Autonomy Test offers guidance in setting limits, and compels the listing of possibilities.

Clearly there is a difficulty with the ranking of dwarfings. Since a dwarfing must be avoided, unless to do it will prevent a worse dwarfing, it must be possible to state in general terms how one thing is worse than another. But how can subjective preferences be assessed in an objective way? Often this cannot be done – people's preferences are not the same. In such cases, the only way forward is to find out, in individual context, what the person wants. This is where the autonomy flip is useful – and where one must respect the liberty of other people. Where the autonomy flip cannot occur, great care must be taken that clearly avoidable dwarfings do not happen – and this judgement must rest on a deeper analysis and weighing of the potential and probable harms.

Exercise

Re-read **The Operation** (see p. xlii of the **Introduction to the Second Edition**). Imagine that you are the surgeon: (a) during the initial consultation; and (b) as he meets the patient on the morning of the operation. Use the Autonomy Test and base a moral policy on its results.

Respect autonomy (brief explanation)

The requirement to respect autonomy is also part of the core rationale of health work, but as we have seen is significantly different from the necessity to create autonomy. The creation of autonomy requires the provision of the physical and mental wherewithal for enhanced movement in life, whereas respecting autonomy requires that the person's chosen direction should be respected, whether or not the health worker approves of it.

This idea is bedevilled with controversy. Many of the really hard cases in medical ethics hinge upon whether or not 'respect autonomy' should be invoked. Some of these controversies can be settled with intelligent use of the grid, but there are no binding guidelines about how far personal (or group) autonomy ought to be respected. A strong (though not immutable) reason not to respect autonomy arises when the autonomous decision will harm other people. Beyond this, the issues must be resolved by personal judgement and comprehensive and appropriate moral reasoning.

Respect persons equally

The requirement to respect persons equally when working for health follows from the requirement to create and respect autonomy in everyone. We regard people as valuable not only because of what each can do, but because of what each is. The cardinal aspects of personhood – being able to value one's life and having the potential for future choices – are shared equally by all persons.

The extent to which the box 'respect persons equally' should be employed is a matter of judgement. However, as with the other blue boxes, if this box is to be superseded firmly convincing reasons are required. If persons are not respected equally, perhaps because resources are scarce, then this is discrimination between beings who are fundamentally equal. If such discrimination is condoned by a health service for unjustifiable reasons then there are dangerous implications for that society as a whole. If it is all right for a health service to discriminate on grounds of age, race and economic worth, then other social institutions have carte blanche to do the same.

Serve needs first

This element of the core provides a grounding for the other three. It gains its authority first from the fact that a true health service must – before any other task – provide for the basic needs of all it seeks to serve, and second from an underpinning association between work for health and justice as fairness. Since those who have made a commitment to work for health are obliged to create autonomy and treat persons with equal respect it follows that they must also want to ensure that everyone's basic needs are met. So, if there are people who have no shelter, or no food, or no purpose in life, or a very limited general education, while in the same society there are people whose material wants are being over-fulfilled then this is a system in which full health is not being achieved. It is a system in which there is a lower degree of morality than there otherwise might be.

All human beings have needs that are part of a shared human condition. Though they are never absolute,[92] they may be said to be factual. Rights vary over history and between contexts, and although it is argued by some that through hard work some people deserve more benefits in life than those who do not work so hard, it seems fundamentally unjust for such rewards to be enjoyed at the expense of basic human needs (though it must be admitted that despite millennia of philosophical labour, no-one has yet succeeded in demonstrating that this is *necessarily* so.[24]

But what is so important about medicine and health work is that this principle has so often been followed in practice. In wartime medics do not (or should not if they are health workers) treat only the wounded from their army, and medical treatment is commonly offered to criminals regardless of what crime they have committed. Within health work it seems there is an elemental humanising principle at work. While some pains and some diseases may be socially caused and avoidable, many are not. A person unlucky enough to become unwell needs help and needs it unconditionally. When it is so given it is a pure moral donation – a giving based on sympathy and a desire to create better possibilities for others. By contrast, if a hospital turns away one person with a broken leg whilst admitting another, on the ground that the first person is a bank robber and the second a bank manager, genuine health workers have no difficulty in recognising that the action of the hospital is morally superficial (in my view).

Summary

See Figure 44.

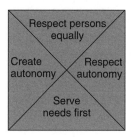

Figure 44 The blue boxes (this figure also appears in the colour plate section between pages 164 and 165)

A review

Why are these boxes core?

The devil's advocate speaks again

> All that is going on in this writing about health and ethics is a cleverish word game based on a set of improvable assumptions that you take for granted. You have decided what health is, and now, by the use of sophistry more than anything else, you attempt to deceive us into thinking that you are uncovering truths. But you are doing nothing of the sort. You are not a detective, you are an inventor. In order to defeat your position one need only refuse to accept

your assumptions and make alternative ones instead – perhaps premises more acceptable to a person of a different political persuasion. For instance, one might just as well include these (or any other) boxes within the core 'health rationale': manipulate clients, create dependency, discriminate between individuals according to their social worth, and act to provide a service for those who, through their own efforts, can pay for it, and do so before you pay any attention to the worthless needy.

Harsh words, but they are from an exasperating devil's advocate who has not understood the argument of this book (and companion texts).[8,24] The point of these works is to provide a firm theoretical footing for a true health service, a health service that aims as its first priority to increase the degree of morality in the world through the interventions made in the name of health. It is undeniable that assumptions about what a 'true health service' is are just that – assumptions. They are preferences and cannot be empirically shown to define work for health. But on the other hand there is a rich and varied set of reasons behind them. These reasons are connected as threads in a tapestry. They begin and end in different places, but link together to present a compelling picture. Some of the threads the devil's advocate should see stitched together are:

1 It has been shown that work for health has a common factor – namely the removal of obstacles to people's biological and intellectual potentials.
2 The associated ideas of 'enablement', 'personhood', and 'enhancing potential' are: (a) richer, more coherent and logically sound than the speculative alternatives of the advocate; and (b) more likely to produce benefits that can be shared by all than any other option.
3 There is a clear relationship between ethics and health, demonstrated in these pages and elsewhere.
4 Certain actions can be considered to be immoral because they dwarf gratuitously. Those features vulnerable to the most serious dwarfing are precisely those that provide the basis for the equal treatment of persons.
5 The existing rationale of health work – in theory and in practice – cannot be ignored. Although things could be better and priorities reassessed, study of present health work practice shows that the principles outlined in the blue layer are already those that inspire much work in the name of health. The seeds of Paradigm Y are already sown in Paradigm X.
6 The practical consequences are dreadful. How could a health service be organised according to the principles listed by the devil's advocate? Such a service would not be a legitimate health service because although it would seek to remove some obstacles to some potentials it would not do for all people equally, and some of the potentials – if achieved – would be debilitating, not enhancing.

Note before moving on that in all but the most exceptional cases at least one blue box should be used during deliberations. A decision to ignore all four needs a massive justification. It is usually impossible to work for health without invoking a blue box.

In other words, though I accept that I personally value the foundations theory of health and my Ethics B, I also think there is a strong conceptual, moral and practical case that other people should be similarly persuaded.

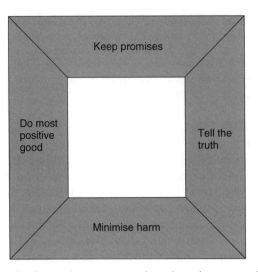

Figure 45 The red boxes (this figure also appears in the colour plate section between pages 164 and 165)

The red layer

This level of the grid focuses on duties and motive (see Figure 45).

What is the significance of this layer?

The red layer corresponds with deontological outlooks, and contrasts with the green, consequentialist layer. It is meant to encourage consideration of obligations other than those immediately implied by a commitment to health work. The duties shown are not the only ones possible (not killing, not causing unnecessary pain, being compassionate and taking due care are some of the alternatives) but are probably the most commonly recognised amongst health workers. Nor are these duties meant to be binding. They should never be dispensed with casually, but from time to time situations will occur where it is better that they are temporarily disregarded and excluded from use. When thinking about health work interventions it is important to bring moral obligations to mind and if one, more, or even all are to be disregarded then very good reasons must be advanced in justification.

The green layer

The green layer divides consequentialism into four key aspects in order to focus attention on outcomes of proposed interventions, and to encourage moral reasoners to clarify their priorities. Ethical confusions commonly arise between health professionals because they have failed to agree who 'the patient' is. It is often assumed that one's own target of concern is the same as everyone else's, when this is not so (see the **Introduction to the Third Edition**). In the same case a nurse may be seeking to maximise benefit for an individual, a social worker may see the family as the unit of care, a doctor may want to maximise benefit for all her patients, and so on. If these matters are not spelt out, needless tensions can be created. Attention to the green layer will promote reflection about whether benefit (which must be discussed and specified in advance) should be increased for humanity as a whole, for a particular group (perhaps a disadvantaged group such as the handicapped, members of the black community, people living in a particular housing estate), for an individual, or for the agent herself.

As with the other layers – and indeed the whole Grid – nothing is clear-cut. It may be that all the boxes of the green layer can be brought into play, or that only some can be used while others lie redundant, or it may be that a box will have to be chosen at the expense of other boxes (see Figure 46).

For example, when considering an intervention it might be concluded that the interests of a particular group might have to be sacrificed in the interest of an increase in social good. So it might be that renal physicians and patient groups get together to decide on the best use of scarce dialysis machines and kidneys, and in so doing agree a ranking of potential beneficiaries from 'essential' to 'inappropriate'. As they do this they will inevitably arbitrate in favour of the youngest and strongest recipients – placing the interests of a particular group (the oldest and sickest) as a lower priority.

Figure 46 The green boxes (this figure also appears in the colour plate section between pages 164 and 165)

But this is not necessarily the fairest or most morally desirable decision, and the green layer should be used only in conjunction with the grid as a whole.

The black layer

The black layer is of great importance, yet includes factors often given insufficient attention by moral philosophers. The black layer is the level of external considerations. In many cases, in the hard world we live in, the black layer contains the most important factors (see Figure 47). For instance, it may be that a person's legal right – say, to receive advice or treatment – effectively takes any decision out of the hands of the health worker.

Figure 47 The black boxes (this figure also appears in the colour plate section between pages 164 and 165)

Ethics is not only a matter of deciding on principles, considering duties and reflecting on likely outcomes in the abstract. Ethical intervention takes place in a perpetually uncertain world of limitations. Although it has been shown that law and morality do not necessarily correspond, existing law will have a clear part to play in some deliberations. Professional codes of practice, although sometimes vague and imprecise, may have a bearing on certain interventions, and it is for the health worker to decide when, if ever, these codes provide sufficient advice.

It is also necessary to assess an intervention's degree of risk, in whichever of many possible senses are most relevant. Will physical harm occur? Will there be emotional damage? Is there a danger that an unfortunate precedent will be set? Is there a chance that the proposed intervention will produce unintended consequences? There is an associated demand on the Grid user to try to ensure that whatever intervention is made is carried out with maximum efficiency and effectiveness.

It is also necessary to consider the degree of certainty of the evidence on which the action is to be taken, and to take account of those facts of the matter that are clear and undisputed. Not to do so would, by any standard, be foolish. Moreover, it is important not only to 'respect people' in the abstract, but to ascertain what their wishes are in practice. Since most professional health workers are in a position of some power and status, many clients may be overawed and have decisions imposed on them, even if the imposition is unwitting.

Health workers should in every case try to clarify the wishes of those they are trying to help, and of those other people who care for them and are affected by what happens to them, and should try to help them conceive of their position and choices as plainly and accurately as possible.

Finally, there is an abiding responsibility (implied by the Grid as a whole) on anyone who intervenes in the life of another person to be able to justify all actions by reference to the evidence. Any person who has reasoned morally in a proper fashion will be in an excellent position to do this.

Limit to the Grid

The limit to the Grid is straightforward. It can be used properly only by those who honestly seek to enable people's enhancing potentials. The Ethical Grid can be used legitimately only by those who are consistently opposed to dwarfing, and devoted to the fight against it. It is meant for people committed to the same Ethics B as I am.

The Grid can be used as it is supposed to be only by people who have made a commitment to work for health, and are seeking to do so with integrity. If it is used insincerely, if the grid is employed cynically – merely in order to further personal goals, for instance – then this is not a moral use, even though the outcomes might sometimes be the same as those that result from sincere use.

A claim for the Grid, and what it cannot do

The Ethical Grid is a tool, and nothing more than that. Like a hammer or a screwdriver used competently, it can help make certain tasks easier, but it cannot direct the tasks, nor

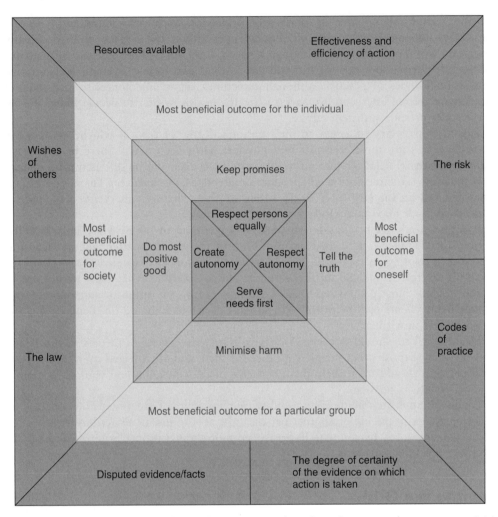

Figure 48 The Ethical Grid (this figure also appears in the colour plate section between pages 164 and 165)

can it help decide which tasks are the most important. The Grid can enhance deliberation – it can throw light into unseen corners and can suggest new avenues of thought – but it is not a substitute for personal judgement. True moral reasoning is an essentially human activity which touches sensitive nerves and exposes emotional frailty. Responsibility lies with the user, not the Grid (see Figure 48).

The limit to the use of the grid is that it should be used honestly to seek to enable people's enhancing potentials.

The Use of the Ethical Grid

Introductions

This chapter explains how to use the Ethical Grid. If you want to use the printed version of the Grid in class, then, like **Chapter Nine**, this is a must-read.

How to use the Ethical Grid

Various uses of the Ethical Grid are possible.[120] Which method to adopt is up to the user, though the following approach is highly recommended.

In general

It is recommended that the Ethical Grid be brought into play at every opportunity (at first even when matters of health are not of central concern). When reading newspapers, watching television documentaries, reading literature, when considering friends' life problems, or when considering one's own responses to difficult situations, it is helpful to practise with the grid to understand its possibilities and limitations.

In practice

1 Consider the issue without reference to the grid. Clarify the issue by identifying key aspects. Attempt to list the pros and cons of the various options for action. Try to imagine possible ramifications. Arrive at an initial position about what ought to be done.

Though it is not a requirement, health workers may find the Rings of Uncertainty (**Chapter Eight**) helpful in this – especially in complicated cases.

2 Express a specific question or state a clear hypothesis.

This is essential to productive use of the Grid – a vaguely focused investigation will fail. The best method is to form a hypothesis – I should do X – based on one's post-clarification response, and then try to show what's wrong with it by use of the Grid. Most users find this psychologically difficult, preferring to search the Grid for 'evidence' to 'confirm' their initial view. But this is a poor use. Given so many levels and aspects it is not difficult to find the reasons one wants. However, the point of the Grid is to enable genuine exploration of both policy and motivation – so it is better to find a way to counter one's biases. If it is found too hard to argue against a favoured hypothesis then the Grid should be surveyed in the company of people likely to disagree.

If the Grid is used in such a group – and it is an ideal vehicle for case conferences and team meetings – it is important to appoint an independent chairperson to take notes, spot inconsistencies, resolve disputes, obtain further evidence, clarify philosophical points and keep the group focused on the Grid's categories. Though this may seem a tall order at first, once the Grid has been used by the same group just a few times it should be possible to rotate the Chair, and so to build up expertise in all members.

The Grid is meant to make moral reasoning explicit. Its most successful use, therefore, is when everyone with an interest in a problem is involved in decision-making. Explicit moral reasoning is public moral reasoning. This means that wherever possible patients – and their supporters if they wish – should be able to use the Grid with other team members. To decide not to involve patients is itself a moral matter, and requires strong justification.

Using the Grid this way will be time-consuming and will require health workers to educate patients to a greater extent than they normally would. However, this is precisely what health workers should be doing anyway – to say it is too difficult, or gets in the way of clinical priorities, or confuses patients, or is only suitable for a certain kind of patient are all Paradigm X excuses. It would not, for instance, be impossibly difficult to prepare a pamphlet for patients on 'Moral issues that may face you and your carers', and explain how to use the Grid in this.

3 Consider the Grid. Either start at the outside and work in (this is the method preferred by most practically disposed people) or begin with the layer that feels most significant. Often a colour or box will seem to leap out as an obvious place to start.
4 Consider all other levels of the Grid. Select – after appropriate weighing and balancing – those boxes that appear to offer the best solution (those that seem most likely to create health – to produce the highest degree of morality).

It is not necessary to consider every box. Their importance varies with each context, and sometimes some are of no relevance. However, it is recommended that novice users reflect on every box – until they become familiar with the Grid procedure.

5 Arrange the boxes 'over' (see the **Introduction to the Second Edition**) the dilemma to check how the solution looks. If the Grid and associated tools have been used well then the problem will have been thoroughly clarified, clear questions and/or hypotheses will have been tested, a range of factors (philosophical, evidential and moral) will have been considered, the process will have been open, it will have been recorded (in writing or on tape), one or more boxes will have been selected – and a reasoned decision will have been made.

Two case studies considered with the use of the Ethical Grid

1 Teaching or caring: Michael and Caroline

Recall Michael, the empathic health visitor assigned an elderly widow as part of his training. Although Caroline did not need nursing Michael visited her for 8 months, and the two became friends. Both were benefiting from the friendship.

When Michael qualified his supervisor assigned him a different case load, even though he was still operating in the same arena. She explained that Caroline's circumstances did not merit the services of a busy, qualified health visitor, and that the old lady had really been useful only as part of Michael's learning experience. Michael accepted this with great reluctance, but responded that he would, in this case, continue to visit Caroline in a private capacity. But his supervisor forbade even this, threatening that it would be a 'very unprofessional' thing to do.

Different thinking

Dennis' thoughts (health worker A)
Two health workers have reviewed the case and arrived at these initial stances.

Dennis feels there is something profoundly wrong about the supervisor's treatment of the pair. It seems to him that Michael and Caroline, in their own ways, both wish to enable each other – not solely as a means of furthering their own self-interests, but in a way that respects the individuality of the other. Dennis suspects the supervisor has a hidden motive. Perhaps she feels that Michael's enthusiastic approach to his work – and his obvious success – poses a threat to her authority, and so she needs to undermine him.

Dennis thinks the following proposal will create the highest degree of morality. Since two people will benefit Michael should ignore the wishes of his supervisor and continue to visit Caroline while at the same time performing a responsible and caring role with his new case load. (Note that Dennis has chosen to focus on Michael's options for action since he sees him as the central character. His *specific question* was 'should Michael continue to visit Caroline?' He might have converted this to the hypothesis: Michael should continue to visit Caroline.)

Mary's thoughts (health worker B)
Mary feels there is something too impulsive about Michael's behaviour, and she also has a 'gut feeling' that the overall interests of Michael's colleagues will not be served by the supervisor approving of Michael's request, or by her turning a blind eye to his visits.

Mary sees Michael and Caroline as mavericks, rebels who unintentionally threaten to disrupt the smooth running of a system that – in the way it operates at present, by rules, codes, hierarchies, and established principles – works to serve the best interests of the community as a whole.

Mary reckons the supervisor is the central character. She thinks the most ethical intervention the supervisor can make is to insist, if necessary in the strongest terms, that Michael obeys her request as behoves a professional.

Mary does not regard this as callous. She takes Michael's feelings (and future as a good health visitor) fully into account – she considers that the supervisor's 'hard line' is in Michael's best interest. The supervisor should, in addition to her reprimand, see to it that Michael receives proper counselling, in-service training, and even career guidance if he cannot bring himself to accept the decision.

Mary has concluded that Caroline is perfectly capable of looking after herself, and should not be a burden on public funds. She believes that neither the public's nor Caroline's interests will be best served by her continuing a relationship that began, and should have remained, as one between health visitor and client. In Mary's opinion prolonging the relationship will be good for neither Caroline nor Michael, neither will it benefit Michael's other clients since it could interfere with his professional responsibilities toward clients in genuine need.

The Grid in use

Now that the key factors have been listed by the health workers concerned the Grid can be brought into service. It may be that it will confirm an initial position, lending it substance and intellectual credibility, or maybe it will lead to a change of mind. Whatever the case, the Grid should be useful.

A possible use of the grid by Mary (health worker B)

Mary, who is honestly seeking to liberate as many enhancing potentials as possible, is drawn immediately to the green layer of the grid. After due reflection on the key factors of the case (which she has listed as 'professional responsibility', 'the public interest', 'respect for authority' and 'the maintenance of codes of practice') she believes the long-term consequences of the supervisor's intervention should be the overriding consideration. She feels that if the supervisor insists on obedience then the consequences for all concerned will be better – Michael especially will benefit – and that the consequences for society as a whole will be better too, because health visiting must be seen to operate according to clear standards.

Using the grid to its correct extent, she considers the other layers. She feels that although Michael and Caroline's respective *autonomies* are *not being respected*, and that by not giving Michael a free hand in his private life *short-term autonomy is not being created*, everyone is being *respected equally* by the supervisor (no exceptions are being made) and *needs are being served first, before wants* (Michael wants to see Caroline but Caroline has no need – Michael's time could be better spent serving the needs of others).

Mary thinks about the red layer and concludes that the *truth is being told*, no *harm* is being done and *positive good* is being produced – at least in the longer term. She carries out a similar analysis within the black layer, and her judgement remains the same.

A possible use of the grid by Dennis (health worker A)

Dennis does not start at the green layer, but with the blue core. His analysis goes like this.

He sets out to consider each blue box in turn, to see how it relates to the case in question. He begins with *create autonomy*, and decides there is no question that the autonomy of both Michael and Caroline is being impeded by the supervisor's decision. The requirement to *create autonomy by removing obstacles from people's physical and intellectual paths*, to enable them to take greater charge of their own destinies, is a foundational feature of health work. The question is: can the impairment of two people's autonomy be justified, either by pointing to greater future autonomy gain, or by showing that the beliefs and wishes of Michael and Caroline are somehow deficient, or both.

In this case the ideas of *creating* and *respecting* autonomy are not far apart. Unless their beliefs can be shown to be clearly mistaken it can hardly be denied that Michael and Caroline's choices are not being respected. As he considers the box *respect persons equally* it becomes clear to Dennis that this is the key consideration. He thinks that neither Michael nor Caroline are being afforded the basic respect due to persons. Caroline in particular is being abused. To use Kant's terminology, she is being used as a means rather than an end. She is not being treated as a person, but as an object. She has been used to train the health visitor. Her personal circumstances and needs are immaterial (indeed they always were to the supervisor), all that was necessary was that somebody was available to allow Michael to develop health visiting experience.

Dennis concludes that Michael is not being respected as a person either. All that seems to matter to the supervisor is that one more efficient, rule-following, functional health visitor has been trained, but Dennis is clear that work for health is not merely work against disease and illness, nor is it work only to create health in a patient (all who are part of an intervention should be considered). With this in mind he decides, provisionally, that the supervisor's action has offended against a vital principle. And, although he has only limited evidence, Dennis also judges it likely that Caroline does have needs which Michael can meet.

Having considered the blue layer, Dennis moves on to the other layers, prepared to reassess his provisional conclusions if necessary. He steps to the black level, the level of external considerations. What laws might come into play? Would the supervisor be legally able to punish Michael if he continued to see Caroline privately? This is unclear. Michael would certainly not be breaking any criminal or civil law, but the supervisor might attempt to initiate internal disciplinary procedures on the ground of 'unprofessional behaviour' – or some other charge she thinks might stick. Would such a course of action be likely? Can it be clearly established that Caroline does, in fact, have needs which justify health visitor support? Or is Michael being self-indulgent? What are the motives and goals of the three people involved? How genuine is Michael? All these matters, Dennis reviews.

After establishing as much as he can about the external circumstances, Dennis surveys the red and green levels, but does not spend too long on these (this time) because the blue core is primary, because the consequences are unpredictable, and whatever they might be, they will not be of significant import except to Michael, Caroline and the supervisor.

Dennis finds that Michael should disobey the supervisor, explaining his reasons, and should continue with his mutually beneficial relationship. He selects the following boxes: *respect persons equally*, *maximise benefit for the patient* and *do most positive good*.

Analysis

Which of the two proposals is the most convincing? Which will produce the highest degree of morality?

Both health workers have deliberated with integrity. Both have used the Grid legitimately, yet they have produced conflicting responses.

A good case can be made out for both responses, however Dennis's position is more in tune with work for health (I think!), and suggests an approach that will increase morality to a higher degree. Of course, this cannot be demonstrated with certainty. As events unfold it might turn out that Mary's proposal would have been more satisfactory. But one can judge only on what seems likely at the time, on what evidence is available and in accordance with whatever moral outlook one has chosen to live by. Because Dennis's proposal shows respect for the individuals involved, because it recommends a genuine attempt to directly enable those concerned (taking into account the likely outcomes in the long term), and because proper attention is paid to the potentials of they key actors rather than reference made to some vague social good (it is not clear how this will be created by the supervisor's hard line – what difference to health visiting as a whole would her tough action really make?). Dennis's proposal appears to produce a higher degree of morality – in direct proportion to the enhancing potentials enabled in Michael and Caroline.

2 Sponsorship and hidden motives

Remember Professor Ronson, the Head of a Department of Community Medicine who wants the department to be involved in as many community research projects as possible, employing as many research staff as possible. The professor would like to embark on a research project to discover why there is a relatively low use of the medical and health facilities in one part of the city. The uptake rate is more or less what one would expect (fairly low because the area in question is the poorest in the district, with the highest levels of unemployment and single-parent families). However, the specific reasons are not known. Taking into account the fact that the local population suffers a disproportionately high level of disease and illness it seems important to understand more about why they act as they do.

Professor Ronson has exhausted his research budget, and has made it known to potential sponsors and research bodies that he wishes to undertake a 2-year project, employing at least one research associate. Unfortunately for the professor, none of the usual sources of funds wishes or is able to help. Out of the blue there has been an offer of sponsorship from a famous tobacco company, which has told Professor Ronson it intends to fund worthwhile health research throughout the country and is pleased to say this is one of its first offers. The professor's dilemma is clear: should he accept sponsorship from a company that trades in a commodity that creates disease and illness?

Another way of expressing this question is to ask: what is the most ethical intervention the professor can make? Although there is no immediate intervention into other people's lives in this case, the repercussions of doing something or nothing are bound to affect others indirectly, and there might eventually be direct and dramatic effects.

Two contrasting thoughts

Penny's thinking (health worker C)

Penny's immediate reaction is that Professor Ronson should not accept the tobacco company's money. To do so, she thinks, would be entirely unprincipled, would undermine the ethos of the health service, would reflect discredit on Professor Ronson and would provide a valuable source of propaganda for the tobacco industry. The tobacco companies would, if their sponsorship were to be accepted, be able to claim they were being endorsed by the health service. Penny thinks that taking the money would be unquestionably wrong.

Charlotte's intuition (health worker D)

Even though Charlotte is aware that many people will feel there is something offensive about a sector of the health service accepting tobacco money, she does not regard this of crucial importance. She thinks about it, and sees there is much to be gained by accepting the sponsorship – many people may benefit if Professor Ronson takes the grant.

After all, Charlotte reflects, the health service is funded from a source that some consider more reprehensible than the tobacco companies. The State (or the government of the day) is by far the largest sponsor of the health service. And much of what the State does undoubtedly harms the health of the population (in a medical sense as well as in other senses). For instance, governments permit industrial pollution, manufacture nuclear weapons, allow people to suffer unemployment when, with alternative policies, they could ensure work for all. Yet very few researchers have any qualms about accepting funds from this source.

The use of the Grid in this case

It falls to each health worker to consider each level of the grid in some order, either to justify her initial thinking or to appreciate the merits of an alternative.

Penny's use of the grid

Penny thinks that if Professor Ronson accepts the money then the balance of good over evil for society will be substantially decreased. Even if there is benefit for the professor, for the research associate, for the university and for the disadvantaged section of the community in question, this will be outweighed by the increased credibility given to the tobacco companies.

Studying the red level she sees that there may be a duty incumbent on the professor to *minimise harm*, and she considers that to accept the offer will, indirectly, lead to harm. Penny is convinced the tobacco company's intent is not altruistic. It is seeking propaganda, and increasingly needs to show it can work for social good to help in its fight against measures to curtail its business. On considering the blue level, Penny reasons that the intervention is too indirect to raise issues of *autonomy*, *respect* and *need*.

Penny thinks the professor should decline the sponsorship, and regards the boxes *minimise harm and maximise benefit for society* of most significance.

Charlotte's use of the grid

Charlotte also begins with the consequences layer, but remains of the view that the good consequences for the professor, the university, the disadvantaged group and the research associate outweigh the possible decrease in social good. After reflecting on the black layer Charlotte reasons that the effect on society is so open to speculation that the outcome of the professor's acceptance of sponsorship can be no more than a matter of opinion. It is just as likely that a fine research project could produce significant nationwide benefits for similar groups of people, and that direct and clear improvements in many people's life quality could result. There is no evidence that accepting the award would lead to more people smoking, nor is it certain that the tobacco company's efforts (whatever its motive) will do anything to prevent legislation against their marketing activities.

Charlotte considers that the 'do most positive good' is the most relevant on the red level, and also thinks the blue core important. She believes that a successful research project could lead to significant improvements in the autonomy of disadvantaged individuals, and will certainly enhance the scope and self-direction of the research associate, while even if there are spin-offs for the tobacco company these will not reduce general levels of autonomy.

In Charlotte's opinion Professor Ronson should accept the money, and denounce smoking at the same time if that is what he wishes. She regards the boxes *create autonomy, maximise benefit for self* and *maximise benefit for a particular group* of greatest significance.

Analysis

In my opinion, the appropriate analysis has already been carried out. For Charlotte's reasons, Professor Ronson should accept the money in order to create a higher degree of morality.

Ten tips for teaching with the Ethical Grid

The Ethical Grid is used widely to teach ethics to health professionals, but is not always employed to its full potential. To use the Grid most effectively a teacher should:

1 Introduce the Grid by *first* explaining its underpinning philosophy of health. Ideally the teacher should outline the foundations theory of health, and build up the four blue boxes as she does so.[24] Once students have grasped the blue boxes' philosophical basis the teacher should add the Grid's outer layers one by one.

2 Allow students time to expose their initial thoughts and prejudices. Explain that the best use of the Grid is to challenge these biases – it is easy to use it unreflectively to confirm them, and this is a danger users should constantly appreciate.

3 Be clear that the best use of the Grid requires a very specific question or hypothesis.

4 Explain how the Grid works, using at least one real life example, before allowing students to work with it themselves.

5 Emphasise that it is the user, not the Grid, who does the analysing. This means that for each case the user must define afresh what each box means (What are the risks? What does benefit mean in this case? Which harm should be minimised? And so on).

6 If using group work, appoint one member of the group as a neutral chairperson, to report back and to keep the others focused on the Grid. A neutral chairperson is also recommended if the Grid is used in teams and case conferences in actual cases.

7 Suggest that the chairperson takes notes of the deliberative process.

8 Note that it is best when first using the Grid to work systematically in, starting with the black layer and ending with the blue. Note too that once students have used the Grid this way a couple of times it is a good idea to ask them to 'home in' on any boxes that seem to 'stand out' for them, as they study the case at hand.

9 If teaching humanities or arts students point out that the Grid is a practical device. Though some of its terms may seem academically unsophisticated this is deliberate – challenge the students to solve practical problems firmly and confidently. If teaching practitioners point out that the Grid is derived from a long-standing academic tradition, and that all its categories are disputable. Allow this type of student to explore the black layer until she feels comfortable with the practical issues, then insist she pays attention to the more theoretical layers.

10 Deal with common misperceptions at the outset. For example:
   i. The Grid can produce conflicting responses to the same issue, but it cannot support *any* answer – at least one blue box should be used in keeping with the foundations theory of health.
   ii. The only relationships between the boxes are the colours. The combinations which make up the 'pyramid sides' are arbitrary.
   iii. Grid users can select as many boxes as they wish, though three or fewer will normally be adequate. There is no obligation to select one of each colour. More than one of each colour can be chosen if desired.
   iv. *Create autonomy* is most definitely not the same as *respect autonomy*.

Conclusions

I hope that the Ethical Grid continues to be widely used. But more importantly I hope it is increasingly employed with knowledge of its philosophical background. I hope that as it is used in practice and teaching, more and more users understand that *all* work for health is a moral endeavour – not just bits of it. And as more health workers come to realise this truth – and commit to a substantial, well-articulated theory of health – I hope the new paradigm will finally gain sufficient power to eclipse the old one.

The Values Exchange

Introduction

This chapter describes how the book's original, speculative ideas have evolved into a unique decision support programme called the Values Exchange. If you want to explore the values exchange you can do so for free by going to: www.values-exchange.com.

The chapter also summarises the relationship between the Values Exchange, ethics and rational fields.

The evolution of the Values Exchange

Since 1988 hundreds of health care ethics teachers have used the Ethical Grid to help students think in a structured way. Though not every ethics lecturer enjoys or understands the Grid,[121] many have found it the best teaching option for vocational students since it demystifies ethical reasoning, grounds discussion in real-life situations, and uses jargon-free vocabulary.

However, there is a massive divide between the classroom and the reality of health care practice. In educational settings there is room to think, whereas in practice staff must act quickly, there are pressures to 'follow the leader', and it is often impossible to challenge ingrained practice.

Increasingly aware of the classroom–reality gap, I began to search for a way to add greater practical power to my ideas. I tried to persuade medical schools to adopt regular in-service training centred on the book's methods; I created a wooden version of the Grid to help make ethics learning tactile and grounded; and I considered films, conferences and training alliances with health service partners. But it was obvious that none of these initiatives was ever going to make the difference I was after.

Then, towards the end of 2000, it dawned on me that the visual elements of the Rings of Uncertainty and the Ethical Grid might be converted into interactive software, which people could use at their computer stations. But though this was a move in the right direction, without a database the embryonic software was barely more than an electronic copy of the wooden Grid, and less effective for group teaching.

I had a rethink. I decided I was tinkering – not being passionate enough. If the tools were ever going to get off the ground, I needed to take their development seriously. So I set up a private company (VIDe Ltd.) and began to build a database – at which point a cascade of 'what ifs?' rained down on me.

What if I could create a program capable of doing what I do as a teacher in a small classroom? What if I could get the Grid to prompt and challenge people as they sat and thought in front of their PC screens? And what if such a tool could be available not just to tens but hundreds or even thousands of health workers – students and practitioners – at once? What if the tool could help them share their thinking with others in a safe and constructive way? What if people's ethical thinking could be organised in a much clearer and more meaningful way than could ever be achieved by even the most in-depth classroom discussion? And what if everyone who has taken the trouble to enter their views could explore a range of quantitative and qualitative reports, with nothing whatsoever hidden?

What if service users/patients could also use the system? What if there were sub-programs which triggered alerts when service users and professionals were thinking differently, or when there were communication problems? What if I could find a health authority or two willing to try the system out for real? What if I could persuade a few university health faculties to adopt the software? And what if . . . what if . . . I could begin to have school students engage with the software? What then?

To me, these were staggering thoughts (thankfully they didn't all occur at the same time). At long last I could see that a world of change – inspired by but far surpassing this book – could really be possible.

In 1988 I wrote, with pleasure and at least some justification:

> This book extends a theory about the nature of health into the heart of practice. It is genuinely philosophy applied. And it is long overdue. (**Preface to the First Edition**)

But it was philosophy applied in print only. At the time I had no idea that words could metamorphose into concrete, life-changing applications. But they can. And now – 20 years on – my philosophy has escaped its printed impotence and become the Values Exchange: www.values-exchange.com.

The Values Exchange in 15 steps

The Values Exchange can be explained in 15 steps. It is so straightforward anyone aged 10 and over can use it.[122]

Here's how to do it:

1 To begin, you must register by answering a few personal questions, then sign in. You can be anonymous.

Figure 49

2 Next select a case:

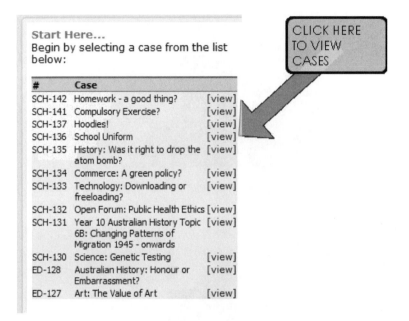

Figure 50

3 Click to respond to the case:

ED-130 – Health Inequalities in Redbridge
Closes October 23, 2008

Many people think that the NHS should treat everyone equally. But if people do not start on an equal footing, treating everyone the same can never reduce health inequalities. To do this it will be necessary to spend MORE on poorer districts - but is this acceptable to all Redbridge residents, wherever they live?

[click here to read background information]

It is proposed that Redbridge PCT will spend more on less well-off districts than better-off districts

Click here to respond to the case in depth

Click here for current status

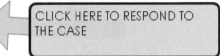

Figure 51

4 Read the case notes. Answer three opening questions. **Tip:** Video Help is excellent.

Figure 52

5 Then click:

Figure 53

6 Write your gut reaction in the free text box:

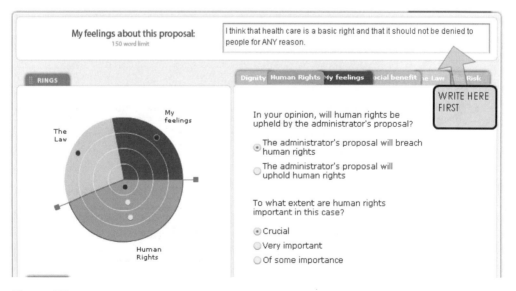

Figure 54

7 Use the wedges of pie that make sense to you – one can be enough. Delete wedges that don't help you say what you want to. Use the free text box to expand if you like:

Figure 55

A typical response looks like this (note how the Rings of Uncertainty have evolved into the Perception Rings):

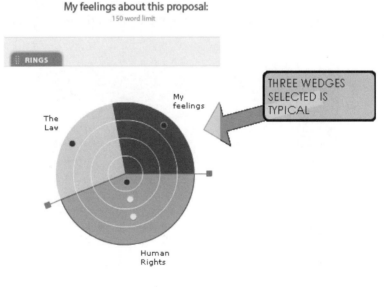

Figure 56

8 Then click:

Figure 57

9 Then either change your focus or just click:

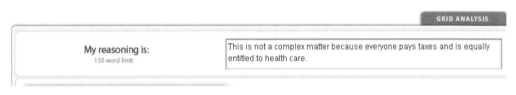

Figure 58

10 Write out what you think should be done in the free text box above the Grid:

GRID ANALYSIS

| My reasoning is: | This is not a complex matter because everyone pays taxes and is equally |
| 150 word limit | entitled to health care. |

Figure 59

11 Click on the grey tiles to see your choices – they turn coloured when you choose a meaning option. Use only tiles that support your case – just one can be enough. (Note how the Ethical Grid has changed – it is now three layers rather than four and the central tiles no longer exclusively reflect the foundations theory of health.)

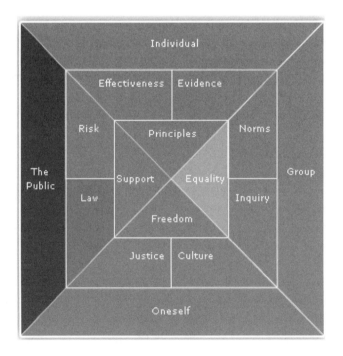

Figure 60

12 Fill in any free text boxes that appear below the Grid:

Figure 61

13 Then click

Figure 62

14 Review and submit. Then explore the fascinating reports.
15 Click the EASY REPORT buttons or use the Reports Wizard for in-depth research:

Figure 63

Figure 64

How the Values Exchange evolved from Ethics: The Heart of Health Care

How the Rings of Uncertainty became the Perception Rings

As **Chapter Eight** explains, the Rings of Uncertainty were originally a sort of reconnaissance device, meant to help decision-makers outline the pros and cons of a situation and picture themselves 'standing' in the Rings. The closer to the centre of the Rings the health worker saw herself for each segment, the more certain she would be about how to act. For example:

Dr Wilson is a consultant paediatrician facing an unpleasant problem. He is responsible for the care of a severely handicapped neonate – a week-old infant. The baby has an inoperable condition but, with prolonged intensive care, stands a 50% chance of surviving, for a few years at least. However, it is likely that his distress – both mental and physical – will be so great that many people would not judge his life to be worth living. The baby's parents – both Catholic – are desperately distressed.

How can Dr Wilson perceive his position? How is he to determine his proper role in this case? What should limit his practice?

Clearly there are several considerations, potential limits and possible courses of action in play. Not all the options will be of the same merit, but he might choose more than one.

Dr Wilson begins to explore the Rings. Logically enough he begins in the competence segment. Now, if Dr Wilson sees himself standing outside the Rings – where he has no special skill or knowledge – he should stop his deliberation at this initial thought. If he is not competent to make the decision he should pass the problem over to someone else, or to a team of people. Perhaps a nurse, a priest, a philosopher or the parents will be better equipped to make the best decision.

In fact Dr Wilson is not so unassuming. He tentatively places himself within the second circle from the centre (B), thus acknowledging that others are expert too. (see **Chapter Eight**)

The Values Exchange's Perception Rings fulfil a similar preliminary function, though users are no longer asked to 'picture themselves'. Instead they are asked to feel a gut reaction, and to select only those wedges that really resonate with them.

Most of the wedge meanings have changed too, through trial and error as the software has developed.

Using the Perception Rings – rather than the older, paper-based Rings of Uncertainty – Dr Wilson should be able to understand his human response more freely and immediately. Since his sense is that the baby should not be treated, he might select 'my emotion'; 'my role'; 'dignity' and perhaps 'the law', perhaps like this:

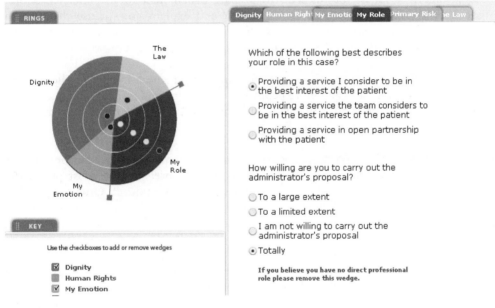

Figure 65

How the Ethical Grid became the Values Grid

To use the original Grid, people were encouraged to:

1 Consider practical problems and identify key aspects. List the pros and cons of the various options for action, try to imagine possible ramifications and arrive at an initial position about what ought to be done. *The same effect is achieved by the Values Exchange, at the **Introduction** and at the **Perception Rings** screens.*
2 They should then express a specific question or state a clear hypothesis. *This is pre-set as 'the administrator's proposal' for respondents on the Values Exchange.*

3 The Grid is meant to make moral reasoning explicit. Its most successful use, therefore, is when everyone with an interest in a problem is involved in decision-making. Explicit moral reasoning is public moral reasoning. This means that wherever possible patients – and their supporters if they wish – should be able to use the Grid with other team members. To decide not to involve patients is itself a moral matter, and requires strong justification.

On the Values Exchange this takes the form either of inviting everyone, or inviting specific groups of people, to reason publicly about an issue. The results are published instantly, and entirely, for everyone to see.

4 Using the Grid this way will be time-consuming and will require health workers to educate patients to a greater extent than they normally would. However, this is precisely what health workers should be doing anyway – to say it is too difficult, or gets in the way of clinical priorities, or confuses patients, or is only suitable for a certain kind of patient are all Paradigm X excuses. It would not, for instance, be impossibly difficult to prepare a pamphlet for patients on 'Moral issues which may face you and your carers', and explain how to use the Grid in this. *Or indeed it would not be impossibly difficult to build a Values Exchange and invite everyone, professional and patient alike, to have their say.*

Unsurprisingly, the same lame excuses for inaction are occasionally levelled at the Values Exchange – yet more and more people are welcoming and using it, and it is getting harder and harder for the powerful elite to prevent people transparently, comprehensively and publicly debating matters of moral concern.

5 Once you have reflected on the proposal/hypothesis you must consider the Grid. Either start at the outside and work in (this is the method preferred by most practically disposed people) or begin with the layer that feels most significant. Often a colour or box will stand out as an obvious place to start.

At the Values Exchange you are invited to click on each of the tiles to view specific choices of meaning, but the process remains essentially the same, as you can see by browsing: www.values-exchange.com.

6 Then keep on reflecting. Consider all other levels of the Grid. Select – after appropriate weighing and balancing – those boxes that appear to offer the best solution.

7 It is not necessary to consider every box. Their importance varies with each context, and sometimes some are of no relevance. However, it is recommended that novice users reflect on every box – until they become familiar with the Grid procedure.

Exactly the same applies at the Values Exchange – only three or four Grid tiles need be used per analysis; however, respondents are encouraged to explore the whole Grid. As they do, the Grid asks them questions – 'Do you really want to say that?' – and also asks them to define ideas – for example, 'What do you mean by 'risk'?' – which might otherwise be left too vague.

8 Arrange the boxes 'over' the dilemma (see the **Introduction to the Second Edition**) to check how the solution looks. If the Grid and associated tools have been used well then the problem will have been thoroughly clarified, clear questions and/or hypotheses will have been tested, a range of factors (philosophical, evidential and moral) will have

been considered, the process will have been open, it will have been recorded (in writing or on tape), one or more boxes will have been selected – and a reasoned decision will have been made. *Far better than writing on paper or recording on tape, the Values Exchange automatically creates a wide range of quantitative and qualitative reports – at least 33 for every single case (Figure 64).*

Ethics, rationality and the Values Exchange – a passionate summary about a piece of logic

Ethics and the Values Exchange

To bring this edition to a close I want to explain how everything fits together.
First, recall what ethics is and is not.

What ethics is not

- Ethics is not a body of knowledge
- Ethics is not law
- Ethics is not rules
- Ethics is not objective – no people, no ethics
- There are no ethics experts – some people can think more efficiently than others, and some people have more experience than others, but no-one has privileged access to the 'right values'
- Ethics committees have no more ethical authority than anyone else
- Codes of Ethics and ethical principles are nothing more than starting points for thinking.

What ethics is

- Ethics is a thought process
- Ethics is personal
- Ethics always involves reflection about a mixture of values and evidence
- Ethics requires commitment
- Choosing what commitment to make is the ultimate challenge for every one of us
- To be ethical in health care requires a commitment to a personal opinion about the point of health work.

These assumptions are the source of the Rings and the Grid, and therefore of the Values Exchange. They are the complete opposite of rules-based, laws-based, principles-based, specific ethical theory-based versions of ethics. These misguided approaches get it wrong because they place the source of ethics outside individuals. They say – read this Code, apply this principle, use this theory rather than that one and lo, you will be ethical. Yes, these interpretations of ethics sometimes invite people to think, but they are basically motivated to tell people what to do – they ask us to think using ideas that are not our own, and which do not emanate from our personal life experience.

Real ethics, by contrast, stems from absorption in life and commitment to a particular way of conducting one's life. Hence the **Perception Rings approach** – see the situation as it appears to you. Don't first look outside yourself for rules or for what other people might think. Picture yourself in that situation. Stand back. Where are you? What is your environment? What pressures are impinging on you? What is restricting your choices? What risks are you facing? How certain is the ground? What are your emotions? What preferences and instincts has this situation brought to your consciousness? See yourself in the situation – as you appear to you and as it appears to you – don't think your answer will be just a matter of reason – it is never just a matter of reason. It is a matter of perception, of you being you fully in that situation.

And hence the **Grid approach** too – now you have confronted the situation as an autonomous person, now you know you are not an ethics expert, now you appreciate the depth of your biases, fears and anxieties, now you have a sense that the situation is essentially a raw, unstructured challenge: you can knowingly apply a structure (the Grid) which might help you think. And – having read this book and having used the Values Exchange – you can apply the Grid knowing that it is a person-made structure, and knowing that you have made a personal choice to use it to deal with your problem.

The best thing about the Grid is that although it is structured, you still have a lot of flexibility in the choices you make – and this is perfectly reflected in the Values Exchange version. Using the Values Grid you can agree strongly or disagree strongly and everything in between, yet use the same choices of meaning. Equally, using the Values Grid two people can both agree strongly with a proposal yet cite completely different reasons for their position. Moreover, one person might agree strongly and the other disagree strongly, yet make the same choices of tile and give the same meanings for each tile.

Ethics is thinking, in the fullest possible self-awareness, about what one might do. Consistency is important, but not as important as genuinely reflecting about what to do as you, at that moment – and being open to the thoughts of others.

It is good to change your mind as you think. Using the Values Exchange it is not uncommon – over the space of a week or so – for people to reverse their positions completely – this is social reality.

The Values Exchange promotes ethical analysis by offering self-awareness and choice – there are no binding principles or rules or laws in it – just the possibility of reflection and learning – about oneself, about the world at large, and about your place in it.

Rational fields and the Values Exchange

Recall the rational field template (see the **Introduction to the Third Edition**). Recall how rational fields seem at first to be solely logical (note I refer to 'the rational field' sometimes as the bubble part only, but it is really the whole thing). This logic is an illusion – this illusion parallels the illusion that ethics is rules-based, laws-based or principles-based. If rationality were only logic then we could never get started on thinking because logic itself cannot select problems for us to solve. Equally, if ethics were only rules, laws or principles we could never get started on ethical analysis, because laws, principles and rules do not select themselves.

Now remember how we can transcend our rational fields to see masses of them simultaneously, and remember too that quite often we can understand their causes. Think about your own rational fields right now. As you do so you create yet another rational field (you thinking about your rational field). This additional rational field gives you a mind's eye view of at least part of the sea of rational fields which constitute yourself and your projects.

Exactly the same thing should happen both when you respond to a case on the Values Exchange and when you see other people's responses to cases on the Values Exchange.

We need never be trapped within any manufactured rational field, so long as we can take this step back (Figures 11 and 12).

If you substitute 'Values Exchange considered responses' for 'rational fields' in the above figures, it is essentially the same phenomenon. As you create a response to a Values Exchange case you create many rational fields. You need only think about what you are doing as a sea of rational fields to appreciate the personal depth of your engagement with a situation.

Inside the rational field's circle/ellipse you are doing the logical stuff – you are following the rules of the Values Exchange system, you are attempting to achieve your goals (finish the case, make sense, be consistent) yet it is outside the logical part of the rational field(s) where the most interesting stuff is going on. Here you respond instinctively (with anxiety, interest, strong feelings about the issue, ambivalence about the issue). Here you bring your values to bear on the case explicitly (this is right, this is wrong, that is unpleasant, I wouldn't do that, and so on). You use a range of classifications that invisibly shape what you think: whether you realise it or not 'mental health', 'patient', 'promote', 'safe' and so on all have limited meanings. You are in an environment – a social context, a physical context, a political context, a work context – all of which restricts and frees you, gives you shape and stops you having shape.

To be properly ethical you need to be aware of these logical and non-logical influences as you are completing a case or viewing other people's responses – only then can you understand the pervasiveness and influence of rational fields.

Imagine what it would be like to be a floating spirit, looking down on the world and yourself, seeing much more than you could see whilst you were alive behind the vision-limiting walls of the logical part of your rational field. If you were a spirit you could see you as you could not see yourself at the time – both the logical and the human aspects of your decision-making would be obvious: oh I see, that's why I made that decision, it wasn't just logic, it was because of my fear of failure, or lack of trust in my colleagues, or my needing to belong to my peer group, or my bad experience as a child, or a current environmental pressure I was not fully acknowledging – now I see my decision as it really was.

And now I know about my own rational fields I can see much more clearly the human reasons why others made the decisions they made.

This is the way to use the Values Exchange. This is the way to conduct ethical analysis – not by applying principles but by standing back from the situation and from oneself in order to view oneself as a rational field and as a person constantly creating rational fields. By doing so:

- You realise that your own thinking is not fixed – you change, your ideas change, your solutions change: this is a fact, it 'just is'
- You understand yourself and others in a deeper way – you understand the sea of rational fields that make up each of us, and the sea of fields that surround us
- You see the relationship between your values, goals and strategies – this is simply what rational fields are
- You see the commonalities between yourself and others – even if they seem to radically disagree with you, they are composed of very similar rational fields to you, and their thinking is mostly like yours too, it only requires one different rational field out of the sea to cause one person to agree strongly and another to disagree strongly
- You see that values and the other non-logical rational field influences shape your logic – not the other way around
- You see that ethics is about you, personally – about your human response and about how you set your goals and your commitment to your goals – what else could it possibly be?

Summary: Ethics the Heart of Health Care, Third Edition

There is no objective ethical standpoint – no laws, no rules, no medical imperatives, no evidence that can possibly compel us to behave in a specific way.

We swim in a sea of ethical processes (thoughts, experiences, compulsions, reasons) and there are no right answers, no ethical touchstone, to be found in this swirling ocean – all we have at bottom is ourselves.

It can be profoundly comforting to believe there are ethical truths, or that there is evidence that can tell us what to do without the need for personal reflection. But it just isn't true.

Instead we are creatures who – when we create plans – create rational fields. These rational fields are not just logic – they are created – as we are created – by history, the environment, by our instincts, by the way we have decided to classify the world, and by our values.

All these features tend to be hidden from us – we often think we are being solely logical, but this is just because we can see the logical stuff more easily – just like we can see the evidence of what a person does more easily than we can see what is going on in her thoughts.

Values are the key. Not ethical theory, Codes of Practice, committees or experts – values are the key because values underlie everything we do. Technical ethics is no answer. People thinking, learning, growing and collaborating in the formulation of social and health policy is as objective as it gets.[123]

When and how will we see the end of Paradigm X?

In 1988 I was optimistic that the end of Paradigm X was in sight. In 1998 I was more realistic; my hopefulness had diminished. In 2008 I know for certain that Paradigm X is deeply embedded in Western culture and will not change even a little bit without one hell of a fight. But, nevertheless, I am much more optimistic that we will eventually move past Paradigm X than I was in 1998 – and this time my optimism is well-founded.

Recall that:

> Paradigm X contains the 'old school' of health care where health is thought to be nothing more than the state of a person not suffering from disease, illness or infirmity; where the medical profession defines its rationale without consulting those whom it seeks to serve; where the idea of medical education is that as many facts as possible should be crammed by students (who soon come to see their 'education' instrumentally – something to be got through to become a doctor); where the idea of providing students with a proper grounding in ethics is seen as pointless – or worse, seen as a threat; where technical decisions are made 'for the good of the patients' without patients' involvement . . . and where measures of success or failure in the care of patients are predominantly quantifiable, emphasising severity of disease, degree of deviation from statistical norms, and life expectancy. (**Chapter One**)

In the space of 2 days, I was recently reminded that Paradigm X is alive and well. I was in Melbourne on business and to give a paper for a colleague at an academic conference, on health law and ethics. My family had travelled with me for a break.

My 8-year-old daughter, Penny, had had a wound the size of a small coin at the back of her knee for 4 or 5 days and as we left we noticed that she had a developed a mirror-image wound where the leg had touched the initial wound as she bent her knee. The next day we noticed that redness and soreness had expanded in patches all over the back of her knee and there were blisters erupting. Obviously she needed treatment of some kind, almost certainly an antibiotic.

Worried, we went to the nearest doctor we could find. We were told we must pay $50 as overseas clients and asked to wait. After a few minutes an unsmiling woman doctor aged about 60 or so, dressed in blue overalls, announced 'Penelope'. The family – my wife and other daughter Charlotte – followed the doctor (we assumed she must be a doctor, she didn't say) into her room. She was brusque and arrogant and asked where we were from, when we said New Zealand she was irritated because she had already decided we were English and was annoyed that her guess was wrong.

She was not reassuring, communicated little and seemed not to accept our account. Instead she decided that the wound was a burn and called in the nurse – the consultation could not have lasted more than 3 minutes. She told the nurse to apply a cream of some kind – not antibacterial – but the nurse suggested a specific burns cream instead – and with that we were shooed to leave with the nurse to the treatment room.

The nurse was more friendly but had no idea what the problem was and said that the doctor had no idea either – which was already painfully obvious. The nurse wanted to apply the cream but we asked her to look at the wound carefully – we took a photograph and explained that since it was not a burn we did not want a burns cream applied. The nurse saw the sense of this and suggested that in that case we should go to the children's hospital.

We did, and after a lengthy wait Penny's problem was properly diagnosed, a swab was taken and she was give a course of antibiotics for cellulitis. Thankfully she was better within a week or so.

Clearly the doctor was incompetent even from the perspective of Paradigm X, but what was appalling to me was that she had no idea whatsoever about the broader purposes she might pursue as a health carer – she could have introduced herself, listened kindly, looked properly, explained her thinking and answered our questions. She could have helped create autonomy in all four of us but instead she treated us as an irritation, therefore causing us to be much sadder, more anxious and more annoyed than we need have been.

The second reminder happened the next day, at the conference. A presenter was giving a paper summarising the results of her PhD research on shared decision-making between doctors and patients with end-stage renal failure.[124] She had discovered that the doctors she had researched were exclusively concerned with what she called 'molecular management' – with clinical concerns about co-morbidity, survival rates, scheduling dialysis according to clinical priorities, and so forth – whereas the patients were concerned about their quality of life – being able to go shopping and to spend time with their families, even if this meant going against some of the clinical priorities. Paradigm X concerns were making Paradigm Y possibilities invisible.

Everyone (apart from the medical establishment, apparently) knows why this is happening: despite everyone else in the world being able to see it as plain as day, doctors do not understand that work for health is work to liberate a broad range of human potentials and so they miss the chance to make health care more humane. They don't miss the chance because they are bad or uncaring people, they miss it because the system that taught them and the system they work in is so overwhelmingly locked into Paradigm X that it blinds them to basic human considerations – and it blinds them to the fact that they need to make a commitment: (a) to working for a specified purpose; and (b) to their own version of what it is to be ethical.

Another way of putting this is to say that the doctors' rational fields are not properly seen by them. They believe they are practising solely evidence-based medicine, but this is impossible – in fact they are stumbling in ethical blindness, unable to see beyond the wall that surrounds their clinical pathways and flow-charts, often almost totally unaware of patients' quite different rational fields. Doctors suffer from both a lack of insight and a lack of outsight.

What did the doctor who first saw Penny think she was doing? What did her rational field look like? Almost certainly she had no idea she was creating and operating in an idiosyncratic rational field, nor did she seem at all aware that the four people in our family were also creating and operating in our own rational fields – her job, in addition to her medical goals, was to try to display, investigate and understand as many rational fields as possible – her own and ours.

The challenge to the members of the medical profession today is not to be less immoral but to be aware of their rational fields – and this can best be achieved by their using the Values Exchange. I can't think of any other way that stands a chance of succeeding, and I admit that the Values Exchange is currently a long-shot too.

Paradigm Y technology is emerging – the answer is not education in ethics, nor even education in the philosophy of health – the answer is to incorporate philosophy concretely and permanently into practice. Then the world will change.

I want to end this book with a plea to all health carers who wish to be ethical:

1 Don't think you will discover how to be ethical by reading books about ethics, not even this one

2 Read books about ethics if you like, but if you find you do not understand the arguments, the jargon or the relevance, do not conclude that you are stupid or that

you are not clever enough to be ethical – conclude instead that the author is not a good enough writer or thinker to explain himself properly

3 Don't try to live according to a single ethical theory – you will only drive yourself bats (and maybe to guilt too, as you try to live by insufficient standards for the everyday world)

4 Do think for yourself

5 Do work out your purpose in life

6 Do work out the practical implications of committing to this purpose

7 Do reflect on your purpose and your commitment from time to time and, if you feel you should, revise it

8 Do keep a record of how you have handled difficult social situations

9 Do consider using the Values Exchange (www.values-exchange.com), because if you do you will be able to achieve these goals, I promise.

Most of all rely on yourself, your ability to think, your ability to learn from experience, your ability to share with and learn from others. Ethics is not 'out there'[125] – it is not the province of so-called ethics experts in fact made stupid by an irrelevant scholarly culture; it is not the province of temporarily powerful people in social authority; it is not the province of lawyers and doctors and politicians – they have no more command of ethics than you or I. Ethics is 'in there' – it is inside – it is in you. And it is up to you to find it, to cherish it, to nurture it, and to apply it whenever you can to make the world just that tiny little bit better.

Ethics is the heart of health care because it lies within the hearts and minds of everyone of us. Just be it.

References

1 Seedhouse, D.F. (1998). *Ethics: The Heart of Health Care*, 2nd edn. John Wiley and Sons, Chichester: p. 47.

2 Seedhouse, D.F. (1998). *Ethics: The Heart of Health Care*, 2nd edn. John Wiley and Sons, Chichester: p. 48.

3 Seedhouse, D.F. (1998). *Ethics: The Heart of Health Care*, 2nd edn. John Wiley and Sons, Chichester: pp. 50–51.

4 http://ashleytreatment.spaces.live.com/PersonalSpace.aspx?_c02_owner=1

5 http://edition.cnn.com/2007/HEALTH/01/11/ashley.ethicist/index.html (accessed 19 March 2008).

6 A Convenient Truth. *The New York Times*, 26 January 2007: http://www.nytimes.com/2007/01/26/opinion/26singer.html?_r=2&th&emc=th&oref=slogin&oref=slogin (accessed 19 March 2008).

7 From: http://www.msnbc.msn.com/id/16472931/ (accessed 19 March 2008).

8 Seedhouse, D.F. (1986). *Health: The Foundations for Achievement*, John Wiley and Sons, Chichester.

9 Damasio, A. (1994). *Descartes' Error*. Grosset/Putnam, New York.

10 An expanded version of this argument can also be found in Seedhouse, D.F. (2005). *Values-Based Decision-Making for the Caring Professions*. Wiley, Chichester.

11 Gail, M., Brinton, L.A., Byar, D.P. *et al.* (1989). Projecting individualized probabilities of developing breast cancer for white females who are being examined annually. *Journal of the National Cancer Institute* 81, 1879–86.

12 Colditz, G.A., Willett, W.C., Hunter, D.J. *et al.* (1993). Family history, age, and risk of breast cancer. Prospective data from the Nurses' Health Study JAMA, 270(3), 338–43. [Published erratum appears in *JAMA* 1993; 270(13), 1548.]

13 Seidman, H., Stellman, S.D., Mushinski, M.H. (1982). A different perspective on breast cancer risk factors: some implications of the nonattributable risk. *Cancer* 32, 301–12.

14 Strax, P. (1987). Mass screening of asymptomatic women. In: Ariel, I.M., Cleary, J. (eds), *Breast Cancer: Diagnosis and Treatment*. McGraw-Hill, New York: pp. 145–51.

15 Seedhouse, D.F. (2002). *Total Health Promotion: Mental Health, Rational Field and the Quest for Autonomy*. John Wiley, Chichester.

16 Jarvie, I.C. (1970). Explaining cargo cults. In *Rationality*, ed. Wilson, B.R. Basil Blackwell, Oxford.

17 Jarvie, I.C., Agassi, J. (1970). The problem of the rationality of magic. In *Rationality*, ed. Wilson, B.R. Basil Blackwell, Oxford.

18 Kekes, I. (1976). *A Justification of Rationality*. State University of New York Press, Albany, NY.

19 Seedhouse, D.F. (1984). Rationality. Unpublished PhD Thesis, Manchester University.

20 Camazine, S. (1992). *Self-organisation in Biological Systems*. Princeton University Press, Princeton, NJ.

21 Gillon, R. (1985). *Philosophical Medical Ethics*. John Wiley and Sons, Chichester.

22 Beauchamp, T., Childress, J. (1989). *Principles of Biomedical Ethics*, 3rd edn. Oxford University Press, New York, Oxford.

23 Johnstone, M.-J. (1994). *Bioethics: A Nursing Perspective*. Harcourt & Brace and Co., Marrickville, NSW.

24 Seedhouse, D.F. (1997). *Health Promotion: Philosophy, Prejudice and Practice*. John Wiley and Sons, Chichester.

25 Seedhouse, D.F. (1998). *Ethics: The Heart of Health Care*, 2nd edn. John Wiley and Sons, Chichester: p. 30.

26 Seedhouse, D.F. (1988). *Ethics: The Heart of Health Care*, 1st edn. John Wiley and Sons, Chichester: p. xiv.

27 Seedhouse, D.F. (1991). *Liberating Medicine*. John Wiley and Sons, Chichester.

28 Kent, G., Delany, L., Hope, T., Grant, V. (independent authors – discussion forum) (1996). Teaching analysis. Informed consent: a case for multidisciplinary teaching. *Health Care Analysis* 4(1), 65–79.

29 Cowley, C. (2004). Medical ethics and law: the core curriculum. *Medical Ethics* 30, 409.

30 Di Stefano, V. (2006). *Holism and Complementary Medicine: Origins and Principles*. Allen & Unwin.

31 http://pespmc1.vub.ac.be/ASC/HOLISM.html (accessed 19 March 2008).

32 Greaves, P. (1979). What is medicine? Towards a philosophical approach. *Journal of Medical Ethics* 5, 29–32.

33 Fulford, K.W.M. (1993). Bioethical blind spots: four flaws in the field of view of traditional bioethics. *Health Care Analysis* 1(2), 155–62.

34 Metcalfe, D. (1989). Teaching communication skills to medical students. In: Seedhouse D., Cribb, A. (eds.) *Changing Ideas in Health Care*. John Wiley and Sons, Chichester.

35 World Health Organization (WHO). (1986). *Ottawa Charter for Health Promotion*. WHO, Geneva.

36 Institute of Medical Ethics. (1987). *Report of a Working Party on the Teaching of Medical Ethics (The Pond Report)*. IME Publications.

37 Hébert, P.C., Meslia, E.M., Dunn, E.V. (1992). Measuring the ethical sensitivity of medical students: a study at the University of Toronto. *Journal of Medical Ethics* 18, 142–7.

38 Seedhouse, D.F. (1991). Against medical ethics: a philosopher's view. *Medical Education* 25(4), 280–2.

39 United Kingdom Central Council for Nursing, Midwifery, and Health Visiting. (1986). Project 2000.

40 Jackson, P. (1995). Processes of persuasion: social interests and total quality in a UK hospital trust. *Health Care Analysis* 3(4), 283–9.

41 Holloway, F. (1996). Community psychiatric care: from libertarianism to coercion. Moral panic and mental health policy in Britain. *Health Care Analysis* 4(3), 235–43.

42 Seedhouse, D.F. (1998). Death's moral sting. *Health Care Analysis* 6(4), 273–6.

43 Loughlin, M. (1996). Rationing, barbarity and the economist's perspective. *Health Care Analysis* 4(2), 146–55.

44 Consensus Statement by Teachers of Medical Ethics. (1998). Teaching medical ethics and law within medical education: a model for the UK core curriculum. *Journal of Medical Ethics* 24, 188–92.

45 Breggin, P. (1994). *Toxic Psychiatry*. St. Martin's Press, New York.

46 Loughlin, M. (1994). The poverty of management. *Health Care Analysis* 2(2), 135–9.

47 New Zealand Ministry of Health (1998). *A Travel Guide for People on the Journeys Towards Equality Respect and Rights of People who Experience Mental Illness.* www.moh.govt.nz (accessed 11 July 2008).

48 Satz, A.B. (1996). Do we really want doctors to be managers? *Health Care Analysis* 4(1), 80–4.

49 Green, J.A. *et al.* (1996). Fair and effective resource allocation in cancer care: uncharted territory? *Health Care Analysis* 4(1), 19–44.

50 Smith, R.S. (1998). All changed, changed utterly. *British Medical Journal* 316, 1917–18.

51 Seedhouse, D.F. (1997). Recovered memory: conflict, confusion and the need to think things through. *Health Care Analysis* 5(2), 93–7.

52 Seedhouse, D.F. (1998). Compulsory in-service training in ethical analysis. Hospital Doctor

53 Kuhn, T.S. (1970). *The Structure of Scientific Revolutions.* University of Chicago Press.

54 Kuhn, T.S. (1977). *The Essential Tension: Selected Studies in Scientific Tradition and Change.* University of Chicago Press.

55 Lakatos, I., Musgrove, A. (1970). *Criticism and the Growth of Knowledge.* Cambridge University Press.

56 Wolf, F.A. (1981). *Taking the Quantum Leap.* Harper and Row.

57 Ellis, W.D. (ed.) (1938). *A Source Book of Gestalt Psychology.* Routledge & Kegan Paul, London.

58 Williams, A. (1995). Economics, QALYs and medical ethics – a health economist's perspective. *Health Care Analysis* 3(3), 221–34.

59 Aristotle (1976). *Ethics* (Trans. Thomson, J.A.K. Introduction by Barnes, J.). Penguin.

60 http://www.archive2.official-documents.co.uk/document/reps/iraq/iraqdossier.pdf (accessed 19 March 2008).

61 McKeown, T. (1979). *The Role of Medicine: Dream, Mirage or Nemesis?* Basil Blackwell, Oxford.

62 Rogers, A., Pilgrim, D., Gust, I., Stone, D., Menzel, P. (independent authors – discussion forum) (1995). The pros and cons of immunisation. *Health Care Analysis* 3(2), 99–107.

63 Brannigan, M. (1996). Designing ethicists. *Health Care Analysis* 4(3), 206–18.

64 Britain's innocent addicts. *Observer*, 28 February 1988.

65 Thompson, E.P. (1985). The transforming power of the cross. In: Bocock R., Thompson, K. (eds.) *Religion and Ideology.* Manchester University Press, Manchester.

66 Katch, F.I., McArdle, W.D. (1983). *Nutrition, Weight Control and Exercise.* Lea and Febiger.

67 Seedhouse, D.F. (1994). AIDS, science and the totem. *Health Care Analysis* 2(4), 273–8.

68 Flanagan, T.J., Longmire, D.R. (1996). *Americans View Crime and Justice: A National Public Opinion Survey.* Sage Publications, Thousand Oaks, CA.

69 BMA. (1984). *The Handbook of Medical Ethics.* British Medical Association, London.

70 Society of Health Education Officers. (1986). *Draft Code of Ethics.*

71 Greenberg-Gold, J.S., Gold, R.S. (1977). *The Health Education Ethics Book.* McGraw-Hill, New York.

72 Ayer, A.J. (1952). *Language, Truth and Logic*, 2nd edn. Dover Publications.

73 Warnock, G.J. (1971). *The Object of Morality.* Methuen, London.

74 Harris, J. (1985). *The Value of Life.* Routledge and Kegan Paul.

75 Locke, J. (1984). *An Essay Concerning Human Understanding.* Oxford University Press, Oxford.

76 Dewy, J. (1920). Reconstruction in Philosophy (1920, New York, New American Library, 1950).

77 Emmet, D. (1979). *The Moral Prism.* Macmillan, London.

78 Warnock, M. (1978). *Ethics Since 1900.* Oxford University Press, Oxford.

79 Kant, I. (1785). *Groundwork of the Metaphysics of Morals* (Trans. Paton, H.J.) Harper Torch Books, 1964.

80 Moore, G.E. *Principia Ethica*. (1903). Cambridge University Press, Cambridge.

81 Mill, J.S. (1910). *Utilitarianism, Liberty and Representative Government*. Dent.

82 Raphael, D.D. (1981). *Moral Philosophy*. Oxford University Press, Oxford.

83 Beauchamp, T., Childress, J. (1979). *Principles of Biomedical Ethics*. Oxford University Press, New York/Oxford.

84 Beauchamp, T.L. (1994). The 'four principles' approach. In: Gillon, R. (ed.) *Principles of Health Care Ethics*. John Wiley and Sons, Chichester.

85 Gillon, R. (ed.) (1994). *Principles of Health Care Ethics*. John Wiley and Sons, Chichester.

86 Beauchamp, T., Childress, J. (2001). *Principles of Biomedical Ethics*, 5th edn. Oxford University Press, Oxford.

87 http://www.lahey.org/NewsPubs/Publications/Ethics/JournalSpring2004/Journal_Spring2004_Feature.asp# (accessed 19 March 2008).

88 Miller, D. (1976). *Social Justice*. Clarendon Press, Oxford.

89 Rawls, J. (1973). *A Theory of Justice*. Oxford University Press, Oxford.

90 Seedhouse, D.F. (1994). *Fortress NHS: A Philosophical Review of the National Health Service*. John Wiley and Sons, Chichester.

91 Sartre, J.P. (2007) *Nausea*. New Directions, New York.

92 Seedhouse, D.F. (1995). The way around health economic's dead end. *Health Care Analysis* 3(3), 205–20.

93 Seedhouse, D.F. (1997). What's the difference between health care ethics, medical ethics and nursing ethics? *Health Care Analysis* 5(4), 267–74.

94 Seedhouse, D.F. (1997). The inescapable prejudice of health economics: a reply to Farrar, Donaldson, Macphee, Walker and Mapp. *Health Care Analysis* 5(4), 310–14.

95 Williams, A. (1985). The value of QALYs. *Health and Social Science Journal* 94(4967) (18 July), 3–4 of Supplement (following p. 904).

96 *The Economist*, 10 January 1987.

97 http://www.archive.official-documents.co.uk/document/welshoff/nhswales/title.htm (accessed 19 March 2008).

98 http://en.wikipedia.org/wiki/Felicific_calculus (accessed 19 March 2008).

99 Mooney, G., Gerard, K., Donaldson, C., Farrar, S. (1992). *Priority Setting in Purchasing: Some Practical Guidelines*. National Association of Health Authorities and Trusts, Birmingham, UK.

100 Koestler, A. (1978). *Janus: A Summing Up*. Hutchinson, London.

101 *Hansard*. House of Lords, 10 November 1987, cols 1350–51.

102 *Bolam v Friern Hospital Management Committee* [1957] 2 All ER 118 [1957] 1 WLR 582.

103 Harrison, B. (1979). *An Introduction to the Philosophy of Language*. Macmillan, London.

104 World Health Organization. (1980). *Mental Disorders: Glossary and Guide to their Classification in Accordance with the Ninth Revision of the International Classification of Diseases*. WHO, Geneva.

105 Koestler, A., Smythies, J.R. (1972). *Beyond Reductionism, New Perspectives in the Life Sciences*. Hutchinson.

106 *Gillick v West Norfolk and Wisbeck Area Health Authority* [1984] 1 All ER 365 per Woolf J; revsd [1985] 1 All ER 533, CA; revsd [1985] 3 All ER 402, HL.

107 DHSS Guidelines (H C (86) 1).

108 Brazier, M. (1987). *Medicine, Patients and the Law*. Penguin.

109 *R v Arthur* (1981).

110 *Re B (a minor)* [1981] 1 WLR 1421.

111 Nowell-Smith, P. (1994). In favour of voluntary euthanasia. In: Gillon, R. (ed.) *Principles of Health Care Ethics*. John Wiley and Sons, Chichester.

112 Beauchamp, T.L., McGullough, L. (1984). *Medical Ethics*. Prentice Hall, Englewood Cliffs, NJ.

113 Seedhouse, D.F., Cribb, A. (1989). *Changing Ideas in Health Care*. John Wiley and Sons, Chichester.

114 Baum, M., Zilkha, K., Houghton, J. (1989). Ethics of clinical research: lessons for the future. *British Medical Journal* **299**, 251–3.

115 Christie, R., Freer, C., Hoffmaster, C.B., Stewart, M.A. (1989). Ethical decision making by British general practitioners. *Journal of the Royal College of General Practitioners* **39**, 448–51.

116 Waldron, J. (ed.) (1984). *Theories of Rights*. Oxford University Press, Oxford.

117 Baum, M. I didn't abuse my patients. *Observer*, 16 October 1988, p. 8.

118 *Guardian*, 4 December 1988.

119 *Guardian*, 9 December 1988.

120 Seedhouse, D.F., Lovett, L. (1992). *Practical Medical Ethics*. John Wiley and Sons, Chichester.

121 http://www.priory.com/ethics.htm.

122 www.knox.values-exchange.co.nz.

123 Surowiecki, J. (2004). *The Wisdom of Crowds*. Random House.

124 Fetherstonhaugh, D. (2007). Shared decision-making: an appropriate model in end-stage renal disease? (ANZIHLE conference 2007, Melbourne, Australia, 28 November–1 December).

125 http://en.wikipedia.org/wiki/The_X-Files (accessed 19 March 2008).

Index

Page numbers in *italics* refer to figures; note that figures are only indicated when they are separated from their text references.